# THE GRAVITY GUIDING SYSTEM®

Robert M. Martin, M.D.

GRAVITY GUIDANCE, INC.
One West California Blvd., Pasadena, CA
ESSENTIAL PUBLISHING CO.
2823 Cumberland Rd., San Marino, Calif.

FIRST EDITION . . . . . . . . . . . . . . . . . . . . . . . . December 1975
Reprinting . . . . . . . . . . . . . . . . . . . . . . . . . . . . . June 1979
Reprinting . . . . . . . . . . . . . . . . . . . . . . . . . . . . February 1981
Reprinting . . . . . . . . . . . . . . . . . . . . . . . . . . . . . .July 1981

FIRST EDITION

Library of Congress Catalog Card Number: 75-11032

Printed in the United States of America
by Ty Wood Printing
1021 N. La Brea, Los Angeles, Ca. 90038

# DEDICATION

To my wife and children who made so many sacrifices to permit preparation and publishing of this book.

The response by letter, phone and visitors from all over the world demands another printing of GRAVITY GUIDING SYSTEM.

The satisfaction, having been found in simplification of fundamentals, leaves no need of a newer or updated edition, but a re-printing for reading and re-reading.

In time a companion book, "Living PRO GRAVITY in a gravitational environment",. . . . .A book that will broaden appreciation for environment's most important member, gravity.

# ACKNOWLEDGEMENTS

I wish to express my deepest appreciation to my many friends and colleagues for their encouragement to write this book. The major inspiration to do so came from the hundreds of patients who expressed their gratitude for their recoveries. These things reinforced in my mind over and over again the need for preparing this book.

I also wish to express my thanks for help in preparation of this book to Harold Hilker, whose editorial advice and help has been invaluable; also to Ms. Marjorie Schlagel, who read the manuscript and assisted in preparation, and to Marie Hilker for typing it. I take this opportunity to thank them.

# INTRODUCTION

Students of gerontology and longevity believe life expectancy of the average human being should be about 150 years. Based on this, the average person is presently living only to middle age of 72 years. Why are we losing all this valuable living time?

As a doctor practicing for many years, I have prescribed treatments and, where necessary, specific kinds of surgery for my patients according to what I had learned in the study of medicine and some of its specialized branches. But with each passing decade, the signs of degeneration in mankind seemed to be appearing earlier. Many of my medical contemporaries are equally distraught, complaining of their inability to "cure" a cold or a simple backache. But through concerted probing into the reasons for this enigma, old concepts provided amazing new insight. Applied anatomy, human physiology, biomechanics, and environment (gravitational influence) now became beneficial agents of prevention and correction.

Being a physician and surgeon who also practices and teaches gymnastics, one discovery became most pronounced to me. I found that my avocation was helping people far more, in many ways, than my vocation. It was something of a miracle to see the wonderful transformation of ailing men and women into persons of commanding physique and stamina; some of these were individuals who at the beginning of their exercise programs seemed most unlikely to improve.

The QUESTION then arose: Why did confrontation exercise work better than operations and medications in many instances?

The ANSWER: Astonishing and yet so simple that one had to ponder why the principles had not been fully appreciated and pursued before. I probed thoroughly into every possible aspect of these new physiological principles and proved without a doubt that they are scientifically sound and medically revolutionizing — resulting in a veritable "fountain of youth" for all ages of suffering humanity.

In this book I will present the common sense means that have logically developed into a most rational system of prevention and correction for an ideal health culture.

In reading this book, you will gain many interesting facts. But if you really want a passport to better health, attractiveness, increased vitality, and possibly a pain-free back, then you will also implement the system of effective stress exchange in your gravitational environment as set forth in this book, *The Gravity Guiding System.*

The customary guidance applies to the physical activities mentioned or described in this book, namely, it is recommended that before entering into any new physical fitness or physical culture program, everyone should first consult with a qualified professional health counselor.

R. Manatt Martin, M.D.
Pasadena, Calif.

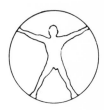

# CONTENTS

| Chapter | | Page |
|---|---|---|

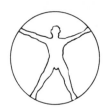

# CHAPTER 1

*Figures... Fallacy... Facts*

O n any one day 8,500,000 Americans are in bed with a backache, and with each passing year, this astronomical figure multiplies. The cost to industry is billions of work hours a year, and insurance companies pay unbelievable amounts in doctor bills and workmen's compensation.

Eighty-three percent of the world's inhabitants will suffer from disabling backache sometime in their lives. Eight out of ten humans will have a crippling backache during their lifetime. Backache has become a catastrophic issue with the insurance companies and with our national economy.

Hundreds of volumes (books, newspapers, magazines, etc.) have been published on backache. Almost all authors of these articles have a single premise: an assumption that low-back pain has plagued mankind ever since man assumed the unanimal like posture of the human when he changed from a quadruped to a biped. They relate that at the time this change occurred, man's neuro-musculo-skeletal mechanism was that of a quadruped, and that as bipeds, our bodies are unable to live compatibly with gravity to this very day. It is declared that because man stands erect, his spine is unstable and gravity has devastating effects—not only on the vertebral column, but also on many other body functions. Thus, gravity is proclaimed to be man's foe.

1

Some doctors contend that medical evidence against gravity, as the cause of backache, is now conclusive. In researching literature on backache, it does not take one long to arrive at the supposedly authoritarian consensus: The primary cause of backache is that the characteristic human erect posture is wrong for our gravitational environment.

These protagonists theorize that life originated in the dark recesses of the earth's seas as a single cell. After eons of time in this state, life presumably became a multi-cellular something-or-other, and in a few million generations, was washed up on the sand bars as a slithering, belly-squirming this-or-that, which in due time grew tetrapodes and pushed its belly off the ground, and thus became a quadruped. Supposedly, in time it grew hoofs . . . and finally claws. With these it clawed its way up the side of a tree where it lived for a few thousand, or million, generations as a brachiating (arm swinging, arm hanging) animal. Then, we are told, this pre-human animal dropped back on the ground as a hybrid, biped, misfit (Man), destined to suffer from backache for the rest of his days because of his unanimal-like posture, with the stress of gravity playing upon a spinal column rather than upon a horizontal spinal beam.

This theory has been accepted lock, stock, and barrel by many in the medical profession; but for them it would

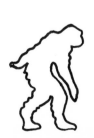 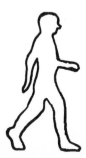

be very awkward, if not downright unprofessional and impractical, to suggest that the backacher walk around on all fours, publicly or otherwise. So-o-o, the prescription becomes one of expediency and substitution: artificial supports, braces, corsets, girdles, screws, jacks, grafts (bone), and as a concluding effort to improve upon Nature's masterpiece — the spine — removal of the intervertebral disc, with little thought about the consequences. *But is this so cut and dried?*

As an inquisitive person delves into the subject of backache, he will find the problem is not so confounding, mystifying, or defeating. He will most likely soon develop some reservation as to whether he can subscribe wholeheartedly to the theory that man, as a primate, has a common ancestry with the quadruped, and that backache is caused by a work of happenstance. All of this, and more conjecture, has compounded the frustration caused by failure of orthodox treatment. *The premise that backache is caused by the unfinished work of evolution is now being profoundly questioned and discredited.*

Every person is most likely familiar with a family member, or a friend, who has experienced one, two, three, four, five or more, back surgeries, and then succumbed to wearing pounds and pounds of back brace with little, if any, results from such treatment and traumatic management. There must be another way . . . a better way!!!

Consider very carefully the probability that man may be a special creation, or at least a progressional development, which by now has removed itself from ancient and ancestral influence. This then demands respectful consideration because of man's own independence, worth, and merit.

As our perspective of comparative anatomy and skeletal-muscular mechanics broadens and matures, the differences, purposes, and functions of the respective

3

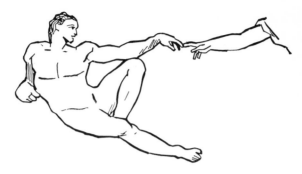

*Detail from the creation of man, Michelangelo.*

structures of man and animal stand out. The results: *We find that, indeed, man is properly designed to live in an upright position.* It then behooves us to consider that there is no connection between the apes and man. Man, after all, is not a monkey! The non-human primate, when used for comparative research to man, is only a model — the next-best thing. The anatomical and physiological differences between animal and man are so discriminatory that some scientific observers have suggested the abandonment of animal experimentation. They believe the need for data adjustment afterwards justifies this consideration. Certainly this is true when attributing man's back troubles to his walking on two legs instead of four. Man, as well as all land animals, lifts himself against the force of gravity at all times. This stress is registered throughout his body by numerous effects. Quadrupeds are not immune to problems similar to those of sedentary humans and are no criterion as to an explanation of man's back difficulties. All land life must cope with the unrelenting gravitational influence towards the earth. *The fact that man can change his postural relationship with respect to gravity is one of his great human attributes.*

Four-legged animals have a head that is forward of the

trunk, sometimes slightly above the shoulders, sometimes lower. The four legs are paired off into front and rear support, with knee joints that either bend backward or outward, unlike the knee and elbow joints in man. The animal spine acts as a bridge between the front and the back legs and as a base for the organs, which are supported in a hammock-like membrane called mesentery.

Although the animal's horizontal, segmented backbone allows for some flexibility, difficulties ensue if too much weight is placed on it. When the spine is horizontal, gravity's pull is distributed over a much greater suspended surface than when it is vertical, as in the upright human posture.

The vulnerable spot of the four-legged animal is its lengthy, segmented back. Constant pressure will deform and distort the backbone, as witness the swayback horse of the buggy age. While it is true that the horse developed a swayback because of the heavy loads it carried, it was still the strong gravitational pull on the underslung body and the weight of the load which caused the spine to sway.

Quadrupeds have serious illnesses of the backbone. This is true not only of the sensitive long spine of the giraffe but also of such strong animals as the tiger and leopard; and the back troubles of the long-backed Dachshund are well known. The quadruped's backbone can be likened to a bridge supported by two legs at both ends, with the suspended part of the bridge broken up into segments and fastened together with flexible joints. This simulates the segmented parts of the spine (vetebrae), held together by the pliable intervertebral discs, with the spine spanning the distance between the fore and hind supports.

There are types of animals that have anatomical resemblance to man and yet have vital differences. These include the monkey and the ape, which we sometimes jokingly refer to as our progenitors. Whether a person believes that he had subhuman ancestry or that he came into being as a divine and crowning act of creation, he can still see that these creatures are somewhat similar in design to human beings. This brings us to the question of which is more anatomically and physiologically satisfactory for man: *The horizontal spinal beam or the vertical spinal column?*

The backbone of the truly horizontal animal, such as the cow or horse, or the semi-erect backbone of the brachiating ape has functional limitations which are considerably different from that of the human spine. The facets are weightbearing in the animal, whereas they are rotational limiters in the vertical human spinal column. In the human spine the intervertebral discs are weight-bearing shock absorbers in the truest sense of mechanics. This is not so in the spinal beam of the animal.

One great difference is that the horizontal or semi-erect animals can only poorly mimic humans, but humans can mimic the postures common to animals. Think about this!

Your ability to practice unlimited postures — erect, inverted, flexed, extended, horizontal and brachiated, with the effects of elongation and decompression — gives you means to control the environmental stress of gravity and allows you to achieve a more beautiful form and a healthier body without backache. You are thereby living cum-gravity (with gravity) through making structural adjustments which are unattainable by animals.

A human can, with intelligence, solve the problem of gravity in his environment in a way completely unavailable to four-legged animals or apes. The force of gravity on his backbone is not along the horizontal length, but instead is compression on a column when he is sitting or standing. His vertebrae, with the respective intervertebral discs, perform better in a flexible, vertical column than when acting as a movable, segmented, horizontal structure like that of the quadruped's spine.

It is precisely this system of intricately shaped vertebrae and intervertebral discs, and the design of muscles and ligaments that allows a human being to stand erect. No animal can stand and move normally in such a fashion. If we closely examine the discs of the vertebrae of both human beings and animals, we come face-to-face with these startling questions: Is it not possible that the spinal column of man is basically more adapted for vertical weight bearing than for horizontal weight carriage? Did man really originate as a four-legged animal as many anthropologists and biologists say?

The human posture is not a biological oddity. Your backbone, like that of all mankind, is best suited for a dominant vertical posture. In the erect posture man has the maximum freedom of movement from which he can take a very large variety of antagonistic postures — postures which maintain symmetrical balance and develop the greatest freedom of action, manipulation, adjustment, growth, and change. Man is not restricted by the horizontal position of the trunk as is characteristic of animals. In addition to his unique ability to walk or stand for long periods of time, man can swing by his arms or legs (brachiate), sail through the air, or swim with the fish. There are those of mankind who have more endurance than a beast of burden. The superiority of a Chinese Coolie or an Indian Sherpa over a horse cannot be doubted, nor can the superiority be doubted of the Andean-Indian who carries several hundred pounds while his llama politely lies down if its load exceeds a hundred pounds.

Of great importance to man are his great strength and endurance under conditions of flexible postural variety, all of which his human backbone permits. He is compelled

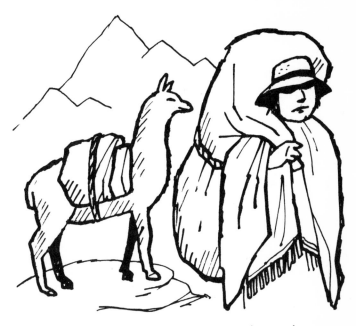

to live in a potentially backache-producing environment of relentless, unidirectional gravity. However, through his ability to employ postural variety, he can live successfully and comfortably in such an environment. *Planned and properly guided postural exchange is the prime tool for prevention and correction of common backache and many, many other physical problems.* The dominant erect posture of the human being should not be considered to be the cause of common backache.

In conjunction with man's prerogative to stand erect, his human mind is capable of acquiring knowledge with which to direct the operation of his body according to established laws of Nature. Man, unlike the monkey or ape, has a most comprehensive mind with which to direct his body to meet its complex needs. Intelligence enables man to fully utilize his great freedom of postural exchange to best advantage. Thus man can utilize Nature's law of gravity for prevention and correction of the common backache, and other maladys.

In some scientific circles it is assumed that the quad-ruped is our primitive predecessor and that therefore its spinal beam has a postural advantage over that of the human spinal column. Actually, it is highly probable that Nature protects the unintelligent animal against the hazards of a human-like posture in a gravitational environment by limiting the animal's postures to that of the horizontal beam. The animal does not have the ideal posture of man, but instead has a most neutral posture. Under this arrangement, the ignorant animal does not require the sophisticated postural management which the human body requires for its dominant erect posture. For example, whenever the ape attempts a semi-erect posture a lesson in innate management is seen. It counters the effects of compression through the long axis of the body by hanging (brachiating) by its upper limbs. By such natural practice of postural exchange, correction of the effects of compression are managed. Nature thus safeguards the animal against the adverse effects of gravitational compression by elongating and decompressing the body through the act of brachiation (hanging).

Man also has the most efficient anatomical arrangement

of the knee joint required to support his body upright. Apes and monkeys must rely on muscle contracture to maintain the semi-upright position; so they tire rapidly. Man can stand at attention for hours, while the ape would become exhausted long before the command of change. In human anatomical makeup, the leg and thigh are encased in tough stockings of fibrous tissue which hold the muscles tightly, and thus assist the carriage. Animals do not have these human anatomical advantages.

Thus it is quite possible that because of lack of understanding, misinterpretation, and circumstantial viewing, the care and treatment of your common backache has been lost in a theory that has become popular and most expensive — not only to your needs, but also to humanity's well-being.

We will now describe new concepts, new approaches, and new developments in treatment of common backache and improvement of general health, which have resulted from an extended, comprehensive study of the effects of gravity on the human body.

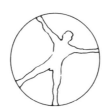

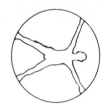

# CHAPTER 2

## *New Concept — Gravity Is Not a Villain*

Gravity is a force acting at all times upon every object on this earth, including the human body. Gravity does only one thing, and that is to constantly pull all things toward the earth. Unidirectional gravity is, therefore, guiding the direction of all weight and forming the stress lines to that point. With the human body being limited during occupation, recreation, and rest to the postures of sitting, standing and lying, the force of gravity can do only one thing to the human body and that is to pull the tissues and organs of the body downward. Eventually this distorts the shape of the body. This is self-evident in the spread of the middle-aged and in the compressed oldster. It should make intelligent people recognize the urgent need for varying the position of the body, at intervals of time, relative to the constant force of gravity.

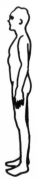 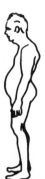 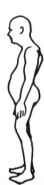

Examples of the consequences of not living compatibly with gravity and Newtonian Law are found everywhere. One needs only to look at his neighbor and his drooping, shortening, sagging stature; bulged out mid-section, and unsightly posterior to see the devastating effects of gravity, illustrating how important it is to live compatibly with this major environmental influence. Too many of us are models of molding tissue living without concern for gravity's guiding power — a power we must learn to respect and use positively. The body is not only molded by the force of gravity but it is conditioned by it. Gravity has been cast in the role of a villain instead of being seen in its proper light, namely, a servant of mankind. It is the limiting of motion and fixation of posture that allows the force of gravity to warp the body and thus cause common backache.

Gravity applies its constant, relentless force to the pliable, moldable, movable structures of the body, much like a potter manipulates and molds clay. The resulting shape depends on how the force is allowed to apply. In both cases, to produce a shape and form of beauty, intelligent application of force is required.

The results of a constant, uncontrolled force of nature on living things are dramatically illustrated elsewhere. Many of you have seen the grotesque, bent-over shapes of trees along the seacoast where the wind blows against them almost constantly in one direction—for instance, the trees on Cypress Point in California. If these same trees could have been planted in large containers and rotated with respect to the constant force of the wind in a controlled manner, they could have been shaped by the wind into normal, healthy trees. In a very similar manner, the form and health of your body can be shaped advantageously by gravity. Gravitational force is a powerful tool and, if intelligently used, will direct its force against the moving, mobile and pliable material of your body in a

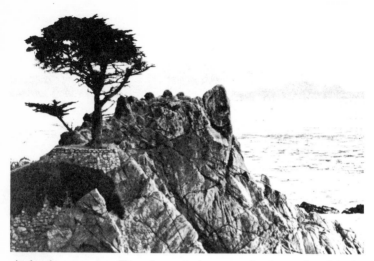

desired manner. The knowledge required to do this is an intelligent understanding of human postures and the influence of gravity on them. By altering and adjusting the postures of the body with respect to gravity, one can guide and control the application of gravity's molding force in such manner as to produce a design of health, beauty, and a pain-free back.

In the ensuing chapters, we intend to show you how to do this and how, through controlled exchange of postures, the stress lines of gravity in the back, the cell walls, the organs, and the whole body can be altered or reversed to relieve and neutralize areas of stress and attrition.

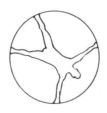

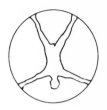

# CHAPTER 3

## *Man Must Obey Nature's Rules*

For example: The setting fowl rotates her eggs methodically, not only to evenly distribute the heat from her body to the eggs, but also to permit gravity—a dominant force vector—to affect the developing structures of the embryo from every possible direction. This action prevents settling, impingement, and fixation from taking place on these delicate tissues. If this were to occur, crooked necks, club feet, and many other types of deformities could develop. The great influence of gravity on the development of posture is observantly demonstrated at the large commercial hatcheries, which stringently meet this change-of-position requirement of nature. In these institutions, thousands of eggs are placed on grids, which are moved by gears that are actuated by clocks at specified intervals. Postural exchange for the newly developing mass, relative to gravity, is an absolute necessity for normal development.

Incubation of the human embryo is no exception to this requirement. The human embryo is well insulated from most all outside influence except that of gravity. This necessitates that the forming body be totally mobile — free floating,

14

gyrating, and free to kick itself into every possible stress position — until late in the last tri-mester of human pregnancy. The developing child's head is then caught in the pelvic ring of the mother's anatomy, posturing the future infant's body in the inverted position. In this posture, gravity's influence is accentuated by the inverted "downhill" pull on the oxygen and nourishment laden blood, which is being forced into the brain to accelerate development by the time of birth.

In the beginning, the individual cell is rotund and hydrated. Therefore, the cell, organ, or unit as a whole, such as the body of a baby, is often spoken of as being round and roly poly. But as gravity is later applied under conditions of limited posture (sitting, standing, and lying), the form of these cells flattens and becomes irregular and ill shaped, with wrinkles and indentations. This is the pattern of the average sedentary person.

Most people start out with youthful appearing, broad shoulders and small waist, but by 35 years of age, far too many develop narrow shoulders, broad hips, and protruding abdomen. With the procession of time, many of the elderly appear pear shaped. Picturing this, we can easily understand why, after years of gravity pull through mismanagement of posture, the abdomen becomes a "pot belly" and the hips become a "caboose." Is it any wonder humans suffer from backache and bulges? These changes in contour make simple acts, such as bending over to tie shoe strings, breathtaking and burdensome tasks.

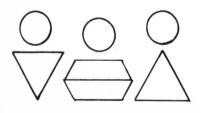 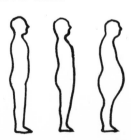

Have you looked into the mirror recently, perhaps a bit wistfully, and found your face sagging downward where it should not, lines traced where no smile or frown could be responsible, your shoulders and chest drooping, your arms flabby? These, and more, are the designs resulting from gravity's uncontrolled effect upon a yielding body which has been in stationary postures, more or

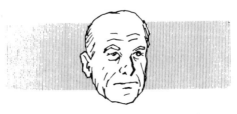

less. You can see that all the contours of your face; all the muscles of your shoulders, back and abdomen; and all your organs, tissues, and bones are exposed to the earthward pull of gravity every moment of every day. *This should impress you with the need to change your postural relationship with respect to the earth.*

In the development of life on earth, no force is of greater consequence than the force of gravity. *This force, without the intelligent use of exchange of postures, can deform, disable, or even destroy your body.*

The effects of gravity on the body are more than surface or skin deep. Within this organic structure, there are many different systems which are interralated, and all are vitally important. They are directly, or indirectly, affected by gravity to the degree that man has limited his postural exchange and permitted a postural debt to accumulate in his body. The potent relationship between posture of the body and gravity is perhaps most readily demonstrated by the position and configuration of special organ systems, such as, respiratory, circulatory, alimentary, etc. (involve lungs, heart, kidneys, spleen, etc). These vital systems are deposited in repository areas of the body in direct response to the predominant positions of the body relative to the direction of gravity.

Another significant organ is the eye, which is hurried into degenerative change by stagnate posture. An exchange of posture produces evidence of change of stress and resiliency of tissue. For example, the intra-ocular pressure may be 3 to 4 millimeters of mercury higher in the supine than in the erect posture. (This is physiological tissue response to change in postural stress.)

Ophthalmic surgeons turn patients head downward to reposition a detached retina. Sedentary living abuses the eyes through routine, excessive use of certain sets of eye muscles. This practice creates abnormal tension on the globular contour of the eyeball, drawing it out of the required normal shape for good sight, and thus changing the refractory capability of the eye.

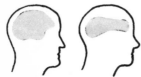 Within the ears are the semi-circular canals which are instruments similar to carpenter levels. There are six of these—three in each ear—placed so they acutely react to any change in the posture of the body. Much of the tottering, doddering, and unsteadiness of old age is due to loss of the equilibrial skills, caused by years of neglected postural exchange. As a result of such neglect,the functional mechanics throughout the body become "rusted out," or impaired, and response to postural exchange is lost. Such postural debt can be avoided by use of brachiation, inversion, and extension exercises.

The organ systems are deposited in their respective canister-like containers: cranial, thoracic, and abdominal cavities. Here response of the tissues can be measured through approximation of the soft tissue content of the respository walls. For example, the brain is originally round, full, and hydrated. It fills the cranial vault with very little dead air space between its surface and the inner surface of the cranium. But as age proceeds and gravity affects a body which has practiced limited postural exchange, the brain becomes flatter and more rectangular. The dead air space becomes greater and greater as the brain settles downward, thus compressing the vital cells, arteries, veins, and lymphatics. The changing shape of the brain also causes an increase in the circumferential pressure. Thus, it has less tolerance for the stress of gravity, which results in loss of memory, acuteness of proprioceptive, and extrasensory response.

Similarly, the *lungs* are housed in the thoracic cage, where they normally fill these cavities, and because of imbalanced postural practices throughout the years, there is diminished tissue response. This results in stasis, congestion, and edema, which cause changes in size, shape and

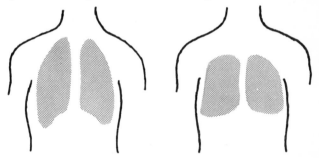

weight of these organs. Measurable differential pressures between the top and bottom of the lungs will verify this. Such conditions force the lungs to settle on their bases, with the apeces pulling out of the cupolas of the chest, and with increased dead-air space developing at the top of these vital organs. It is interesting to note that the site of malignancy in these organs is related to postural embarrassment.

The mechanical function of the heart is remarkably influenced by the musculo-skeletal system. If the posterior muscles of the neck are in proper extension, they will tend to be properly tense. Tensing the muscles and fascia of the front part of the neck will remove their sagginess; lack of tension leads to jowls and double chin. But even more important, the fascia of the neck should be kept firm and in good tone because it is connected to the pericardium of the heart and, in turn, to the diaphragm.

In order to carry a snout and a potted belly the horizontal posture and spinal beam of the quadruped animal may well have advantages over the spinal column of the human being.

There is, however, great advantage to the vertical spinal column of man in whom the face replaces the snout, and in whom the brain is a greater mass which needs support directly under it. The animal's horizontal posture and the ligamental suspension of organs from the segmented, vertical vertebrae makes the "potbelly" quite acceptable and satisfactory for the animal kingdom. The animal's

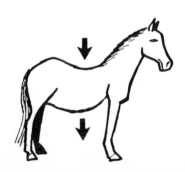

horizontal monoposture and belly-down structure allows, at best, minimal musculo-dynamic function of its torso.

Conversely, in man the weight of the abdominal organs is not carried primarily by the ligamental suspension but instead almost totally by the containing walls. In the quadruped the body is a tube in which support of the organs is provided almost entirely by ligamental suspension, whereas in the biped the tonic rhythmic muscular action of the inverted cone structure of the torso is the force which keeps the viscera (organs) in position. When the human body is placed in the horizontal position the body becomes a tube, not unlike that of the animal, in which the organs tend to hang and fall against the supporting abdominal wall when the body is in the prone (face-down) position, or against the spine when the body is in the supine (face-up) position. Such positions place the horizontal spine so that the stress is on the facets of the vertebrae and not on the intervertebral-disc shock absorbers.

Study of animal anatomy and physiology, as analogous to human structure, has brought to light certain errors in contentions relative to biological similarity of the quadruped to the biped. The belief that ligaments (mesentery) support and suspend the internal organs in man, as in animal, has been disproved by attested and recorded evidence. The soft tissues attached to the spinal column and internal organs of erect man limit motion, that is, right to left or left to right, front to back or back to front. Their function is similar to that of a rope used to tie a boat to the dock — the rope does not keep the boat afloat but keeps it from drifting.

In man the shape of the torso (inverted cone) and the pliability of the walls have the effect on the organs of buoying them up — much like water does a boat. With each breath the muscles lift the inverted cone and its organ contents upward, thus mechanically keeping the organs

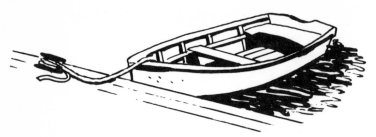

"afloat." The greater the rotundity of the abdomen the less the musculo-dynamics function. The degree of stress placed upon the so-called ligamental tissues by weight load depends directly upon the shape and degree of tone of the inverted abdominal cone. In direct proportion to the loss of musculo-dynamics (loss of abdominal cone shape), organ-fall (ptosis) occurs and attachment tissue becomes suspensional in function. Using the analogy of the boat, it would be as if the water level were to suddenly drop considerably, whereupon the boat would be dangling from the dock by the rope which had previously simply kept it from drifting away. Musculo-dynamics is most highly developed in man with his erect posture and functions most normally when he is at the peak of his postural development.

It has been suggested that if in a healthy body all of the ligaments of the organs were severed they would remain in normal position, and only a straight diverting pull

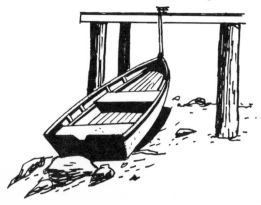

would cause displacement. It has also been stated that all the ligaments in the abdomen are incapable of supporting the weight of the liver alone. This in no way detracts from the fact that ligaments and mesenteries can be trouble-makers and symptom-producers. The attachment tissues, from spine to organ, are traversed by nerve, blood, and lymph channels extending to and from the viscera (organs). The stress and strain of excessive fatigue, caused by limited posture (excessive sitting, standing, and lying), permits gravity's pull to produce devitalizing tension on these tissues. The results are abnormal nerve impulses, abnormal blood circulation, and lymph loss — all of which contribute to susceptibility to disease and to the process of aging. The stress on malpositioned organs inevitably produces malfunction of cells and change in tissue. This, perhaps, is a contributing cause to ailments of mysterious and baffling natures.

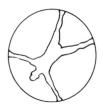

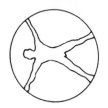

# CHAPTER 4

## *The Torso*

The torso has a great deal to do with making the body beautiful and manageable. When the torso is ideally shaped, it has the figure of an inverted muscular cone (musculo-dynamics). The function of this form is of greater significance than appears on the surface.

The concept of musculo-dynamics portrays the mechanical adjustments which occur in a geometrically designed, flexible, pliable, constantly shaping and reshaping canister (torso). Changes occur in area, volume relationships, hydraulics, supporting angles, and planes, according to the laws of physics. The vectors of stress produced by gravity form patterns in the human body. Bodily function depicts its form; to wit, the narrow waist of the horizontal bar performer, the broad hips of the sitter,

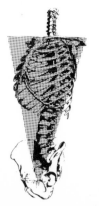

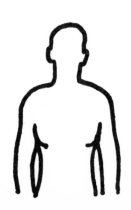

and the straight spine of the contortionist.

The inverted musculo-dynamic cone, which is characteristic of the human, is by mechanical design and function a phenomenon of synergistic forces. The two boney hoops — the rib cage above and the pelvic ring below — are the attachment points of the torso muscles. With the ribcage circumference being greater than that of the pelvic ring, the formation from top to bottom is that of a cone resting on the tapered end. Within this anatomical shape the rhythms of respiration and the abdominal muscles coordinate to provide a buoying effect that keeps the internal organs "afloat." This dynamic action of external muscles supports the internal organs. We have noted that musculo-dynamics functions properly only when the muscles are in good tone. The weakening of these muscles — through disuse and the constant tugging of gravity while functioning in postures that are limited to sitting, standing, and lying — cause the organs to migrate toward the lower and bulged-out end of the cone. This is aided and abetted by the middle-age accumulation of excess fat which overloads the cone abdomen. Consequently, the abdominal wall is broken down, and the elasticity and tonicity of the muscles is lost. The lower part of the cone becomes distended, and the figure becomes pear-shaped. Normal intra-abdominal pressure is interrupted and organs are misplaced. It is apparent that proper intra-abdominal pressure is essential to maintenance of the normal position of viscera (internal organs) in the body. One must emphasize: Intra-abdominal pressure is dependent upon normal tonicity of the muscles of the abdominal cavity, and this can only exist if the natural inverted-cone contour of the muscular torso is present.

Sagging exists in nearly everyone today — youngsters often included — especially in those who have allowed the girth of their waist to expand. The first step toward correction is the will to relocate misplaced organs. Repositioning results in correction of inter-abdominal pressure. Once the organs are back in position, tension is relieved, circulation is normalized, and function is improved. The desire to relocate organs and to correct malpositions is in itself insufficient. There must also be a knowledge of the proper means to relocate the organs for there are both good and bad ways to achieve this.

A most ineffective means for relocation is the surgical procedure of "pinning-up organs by shortening the ligaments." This is a mechanical effort to force the attachment tissues to become permanently suspensory. In the majority of instances, raising fallen abdominal organs by postural correction is better than by surgical operation. The organs in the torso have the advantage of a pliable abdominal wall made of extensible muscle. This wall protects the organs as long as the muscles are strong; yet it allows distension for food storage and, in women, for the growth of a baby. Good posture is synonymous with a cone-like torso. Such a torso constrains stretching of the abdominal organs; stretching of vascular and lymphatic channels; and stretching of mesentery (mesocolon and splanchnic) tissues.

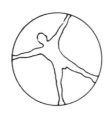

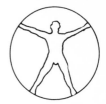

# CHAPTER 5

## *The Spine*

Ⓘn the foetal stage of human development the body must conform to the quarters it is in. This helps to establish the primary flexed curvatures: kyphosis of the dorsal, sacral, and coccygeal portions of the spine. Flexion is the original position of the vertebral column. During the time of the intra-uterine development Nature does her best to protect the embryo from all outside influence.

After the usual head-first entrance into the world the child is commonly placed on a flat-bottomed crib. This should be elevated at the foot-end to deliver the maximum blood supply to the brain and to drain the respiratory tract.

As the child gains strength, it will roll over (face down) and start to raise its heavy head. This causes hyper-tonicity of the extensor muscles of the spine, thereby setting the pattern for the development of the secondary spinal curvatures, which are lordosis of the cervical (neck) and lumbar (lower) spine. These secondary curves are further developed when the child assumes the crawl posture in which the body is suspended like a quadruped, and the spine sags animal-like or swayback-like.

Vertical compression of the body does not begin until the child tries to sit up. The effect of gravitational stress on the body is increased, and the body goes into flexion, as witness the "C" shape of an infant's back when

26

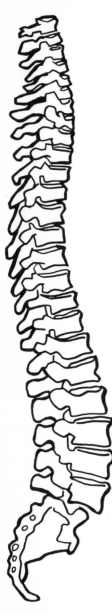

it first attempts the sitting posture. The heavy head falls forward, the back bows into extreme flexion, and the muscles of the neck labor to lift and hold the heavy head erect. In time, the child achieves sufficient spinal and lower limb strength to hazard the squat position. If left alone, it will in its own good time rise up into the regal posture of His Lordship's erect orthostance. Compression, acting through the long axis of the body, causes compensatory curves to be markedly established, and soon the spine becomes "S" shaped, resulting in a beautiful body.

During its posture progression, the infant will, by Nature's directive, be periodically found resting, sleeping, and relaxing in the knees-to-chest posture for hours at a time. Posture, from the moment of birth to that of adolescence, and throughout adult life, continually undergoes molding, tempering, conditioning, and structural adjustment. This, for better or worse, depends on intelligent application of the basic sciences of bio-physics, bio-mechanics, and mechano-therapy.

Human posture is based on scientific principles and not on folklore or erroneous teachings (ancestral heritage, anthropology of posture, etc.).

The human spine is an exceedingly intricate system of bones interspersed with cushion-like shock absorber pads (discs), which form a flexible protective conduit for the spinal portions of the central nervous system. This construction enables the spinal column to move freely while serving as a mechanical support for the entire body.

The horizontal spinal beam of the animal carries the body load on the facets of the vertebrae; therefore, the intervertebral discs cannot serve as efficient load-carrying shock absorbers. Conversely, the human spinal column employs the facets only to limit rotation. The intervertebral discs, whose structural arrangement is designed for load carrying, function as shock absorbers. They aid in disbursement of weight on the broad porch-like body of the vertebrae.

As man devolutes toward the animal-like horizontal posture (dowagers hump, round shoulders, compressed chest, pot belly, off-angle head and neck), irregularities develop in a domino fashion.

As the belly becomes pot shaped, the shoulders round (kyphose) to counter the weight load in front. These changes combine with the effect of a compressed, warped posture, from the top of the head downward, to produce an ever-increasing swayback. In general, the stature shrinks, and the loss of balance between the antagonistic muscle groups reduces their holding strength. The pelvis rotates downward and backward, making the hips appear as a "caboose", since the muscles on the front part of the body shorten — especially the anterior leg muscles.

The body is then in a state of constant strain. The anatomy is now seriously disarranged. With the neck off angle and with the head protruding, there can be many painful symptomatic distortions from top to bottom, such as: headache, neck ache, shoulder ache, backache, chest ache, hip ache, leg ache, etc. Under these conditons, your well-meaning family, neighbor, or relative may rush you off to the orthopaedist, neurosurgeon, or specialist, who will likely place all the blame for your suffering on one or more of the intervertebral discs with the statement, "It is degenerated, ruptured, or protruding, and must be removed." Most likely, at this point, no one has assured you that the discs are not infallibly associated wtih your symptoms. It is deviation from the normal physiological curves of the spine which is primarily responsible for the painful symptoms. Until the physiological health of your spine is restored, you will be subject to continuous or recurrent attacks of pain, even after one or more "scape-goat" discs have been removed on one or more occasions.

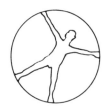

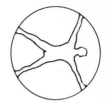

# CHAPTER 6

## *Six Basic Human Postures*

**M**an must recognize that he is distinctly different from the animal and that he is superior to all other forms of known life. He can, to a great degree, control and master his environment. Since he is the only creature capable of acquiring knowledge of his own body structure, he can take advantage of this privilege and use his intelligence to operate his body so as to use the laws of Nature to his advantage. Thus, by changing the position of his body relative to the constant force of gravity he is able to use gravitational force as a stress equalizer. Gravity can then become a great adjuster of his tissues and structures by creating equilibrium through a combination of positions.

In the ordinary, or common, postures, such as sitting or standing, the force of gravity is applied only in compression towards the feet. To reverse or modify the application of this constant force to our body, new and uncommon postures must be learned and used.

A simple example of how the effects of a unidirectional source of energy may be beneficially modified by altering exposure to the direction of this energy is the following: When a chicken is cooked under a broiler only its top surface is exposed to the radiant heat energy, and this surface will tend to become overcooked. But if we place this chicken on a rotating spit then all of its surface will be exposed to the radiant heat, and very different effects will be obtained from this unidirectional source of energy.

In the same manner, we can change the effects of the unidirectional force of gravity on our body by changing its position relative to the direction of gravity, with attending benefits. We do this by varying our posture.

The following tabulation and sketches show the six basic human postures. These are divided into two categories of Common and Uncommon Postures. The physiological effects of each category are shown. Note that the common postures produce compression and shortening of stature while the uncommon postures produce opposite effects, namely, decompression and elongation.

In the following chapter we will discuss each of these postures and describe how the uncommon postures, when properly employed, will counter and correct the damaging effects produced in the body by gravity from exclusive use of the common postures.

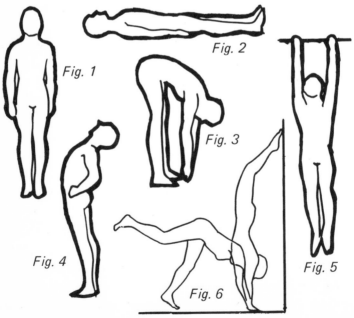

Fig. 1
Fig. 2
Fig. 3
Fig. 4
Fig. 5
Fig. 6

GROUP I — Common Postures

Effects: Produce body compression and shortening of stature.

Used: In work, play, rest, etc.

1. The ERECT POSTURE (Fig. 1)
   (The posture of Dominance)
   a. Sitting
   b. Standing

2. The HORIZONTAL POSTURE (Fig. 2)
   (The posture of neutrality)
   a. Lying (On side, back, or front)

3. The FLEXED POSTURE (Fig. 3)
   (The posture of Accessibility)
   a. Bending forward

GROUP II — Uncommon Postures

Effects: Produce body decompression and elongation of stature.

Used: To counter and correct adverse effects of gravity produced by the common postures

4. The EXTENDED POSTURE (Fig. 4)
   (The posture of Bending Backwards)

5. The BRACHIATED POSTURE (Fig. 5)
   (The posture of hanging by the limbs — upper or lower)

6. The INVERTED POSTURE (Fig. 6)
   (The Upside-down Posture)
   a. Standing on the hands
   b. Standing on the forearms
   c. Hanging by the lower limbs

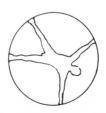

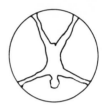

# CHAPTER 7

## *The Erect Posture*

The *Erect Posture* is a heritage unique to man only, and it is his most used posture. It is to the great glory of the human race that its members can ambulate on two legs. "Mark the upright man" — Psalmist.

The average man will spend two-thirds of his life, or 16 hours a day, in the dominant postures of sitting and standing. When you sit there is a much greater load on the spine than when you stand. When you stand on your feet the weight of your body rests on a surface less than one-sixth of the vertical height of the body. The erect body functions by the principle of oppositional balance. It does this so well that there are few perceptible muscular contractions until accumulated fatigue from prolonged sitting and standing cause muscular exhaustion.

When the body is in any of the erect postures the weight of the upper body imposes a force that tends to compress the spine from end to end. The inclinatory effect created by this increases rounding of the shoulders (kyphosis of dorsals), swaying of the lower back (lordosis of the lumbars), curving of scoliosis (lateral curvature), and thinning of the discs (degenerative disc) to a degree that is in direct proportion to the time spent in prolonged sitting and standing.

With sufficient rest and normal health the equilibrium of the body parts is so precise that the antagonistic forces are minimized and muscular efficiency is maintained by the accuracy of bone balanced on bone. The skeletal poise (load carried through the hard tissues) actually supports the body weight. To secure this precise arrangement, three major leveling segments are involved: the feet, the pelvis, and the shoulders. The equilibrium of what lies above each of these respective anatomical structures depends on how leveled and centered they are.

In the ideal erect posture, the pelvis is balanced on the legs; the thoracic cage (chest) is balanced on the pelvis so that the torso forms an inverted cone; and the head is held erect over the chest. Under these conditions, a plumb line dropped from the ear lobe would pass through the shoulder, trunk and femur and touch the floor just in front of the heel.

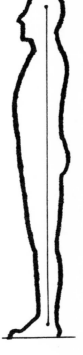

The lower abdomen will be flat, although the upper abdomen will be slightly rounded. For good erect posture, the pelvis will not be tilted forward and downward with the hips protruding in an unsightly manner. Instead, the lower back will be curved in, but this should not be in excess of 10 degrees from the vertical. The upper back will be curved outward in a compensatory manner. The shoulders will be level. The head will be tilted — neither frontward nor backward — but in a commanding, stately position. The spine will be nearly straight when viewed from all directions.

By contrast, let us consider the commonly observed mal-erect posture; a posture which is falsely blamed on gravity and is seen in a great many bipeds walking our streets. The weight is not properly balanced on the respective segmented foundation levels. The abdomen is flabby, atonic, and pendulous — protruding excessively forward over the tilted pelvis. The lower back is curved inward more than 10 degrees to compensate for shoulders that are held in a counter-balanced manner, that is, rounded backwards to offset the "potbelly." The head then is held off angle to counter the maladjusted overcompensation. The chest is flat, thus allowing the ribs to take a position that is nearer than normal to the pelvis, thereby compressing all the internal organs. Changes in the rib cage can cause a decrease in vital capacity, which may eventually lead to cor pulmanale and heart failure.

In fact, the body becomes sunk in from the overtime it spends in the sitting and standing postures. As you reflect on this matter, how much of this applies to your physical condition?

The human body is continually adjusting to the stress of gravity. Whether it can successfully do this to physiological satisfaction depends upon the frequency of postural exchange. Anything can be overdone and being in the erect posture is no exception. If you are an average person with a backache, you have probably abused your *erect posture* by spending your youthful dividends and are now running around with a postural debt, that is, round shoulders, humpback, protruding abdomen, etc. The body's deterioration through misuse of the erect posture is not evidence of constitutional inadequacy of your human biped stance; instead, it is lack of intellectual appreciation of the human postures in a gravitational environment. Altering stress by use of all the human postures greatly limits attrition.

Ability to continue to maintain the ideal erect posture requires physiological and anatomical employment of all the postures to meet the body's different requirements.

When you are in the erect standing posture, the blood has a tendency to accumulate in the legs and dependent parts of your body. Physiologists tell us that one-fourth of the total quantity of blood in the body is in the peripheral circulation, one-fourth is in the heart and lungs, one-fourth is in the liver, and one-fourth is in the remaining viscera. Crowding by poor posture, when on the feet or sitting, burdens the heart, lungs, diaphragm, stomach, liver, gall bladder, pancreas, and small intestines. This stasis causes other chronic conditions.

In the erect posture the heart must pump blood from the soles of the feet to the head through each of the compressed vital organs in the body. This works well as long as compression is followed by decompression. Exchange of postures creates a physiological pumping effect on all the tissues: liquid, semi-liquid, and solid structures of the body.

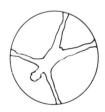

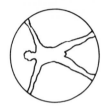

# CHAPTER 8

## *The Horizontal Posture*

The second most-used posture is the horizontal posture. One-third of our lifetime is spent horizontally. We begin our existence in the horizontal position, and every day of our life from then on we resort to this position for rest and relaxation.

Little effort on the part of our muscles is required in this position. Few or no demands are made on the nervous system and the musculo-skeletal structure in maintaining equilibrium. Horizontal is the most neutral of all postures. Circulatory resistance is minimized; therefore, vascular prolapsis is relieved.

Man uses the horizontal posture during his resting hours, and then his spine is supported by the surface on which he lies. In human usage, the spine is seldom used as an unsupported, segmented beam.

The horizontal posture is the most effortless of all postures. Even so, while in this posture, man will change from side to side and front to back to make physiological adjustments. The typical sleeper changes his position about every 7¾ minutes. These motivations for postural change during sleep are indicative of the stress of gravity upon the body. Even while reclining, the effects of gravity continue. Gravity causes congestion of blood, stretched muscles, cramped joints, pressure of the body on the mattress, and pressure of organs on organs.

Research has shown that after a night's rest in a horizontal position the body is taller than after a day's work in an upright position. This demonstrates the need for postural exchange. While lying down, the body's weight is relieved from its vertical compression for six to ten or more hours. Tissue resiliency reflects the recuperative powers of rest. Recuperative capacity is greatest throughout the formative years of life when the body is still in the process of growing. Growth has a lengthening and lifting effect, which is readily observed in the natural development of young people who perform exchange of postures naturally.

However, as years pass, certain capabilities are no longer present, such as the capacity for growth. Thus, as we grow older, we must strive harder to keep in good physical condition and in tune with nature's aims.

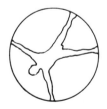

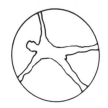

# CHAPTER 9

## *The Flexed Posture*

**D**o not think of either flexion or extension as "pure" posture since they always exist in conjunction with erect (sitting or standing), or horizontal, or brachiating postures. Flexion and extension are attributes uniquely available to the human body while it is in the erect or horizontal posture. In flexion, the body has better access to the benefits of some special senses. Flexion, like exten-sion, can be measured in degrees for grading effect and accomplishment. Normal occupational and recreational activities usually require only partial flexion or partial extension. Moreover, prolonged postures can become a handicap to the body, since they create an imbalance between the antagonistic muscle groups. If overdone, the resulting effect is 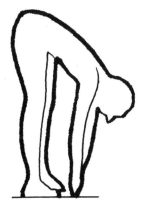 "stiffness of joints." Those suffering from backache have often lost the ability to totally flex or extend the body. Backache is an obvious indication of a mechanically sick spine — one which has lost its elasticity, spontaneity, and resilience.

Shortly after free standing is added to the multi-postural accomplishment of a child, a unique human characteristic, the dominant erect posture, becomes so habitual that downward force of gravity tends to warp the dorsal spine into excessive flexion (round shoulders). This is the beginning of real trouble if permitted to develop beyond that of postural efficiency.

The human body flexes or bends forward readily in absence of a protruding stomach. The slim waist of the torso is one of the human features which makes man especially adapted to achieving the flexed posture.

Man's knees bend forward, rather than backward as they do in many four-legged animals, and elbows bend in a fashion characteristic only to man.

Flexion is a natural continuation of reaching forward and grabbing with the hands. In flexion, the body moves forward from the hips. The muscles of the back are stretched, and the strain on the body is shifted forward to the thigh and abdominal muscles. If an individual does nothing to compensate for this, he is prone to develop a contracted, compressed posture. In either the sitting or standing positions, most people are in a state of partial flexion. In fact, poor posture — whether by sitting or standing — is usually the result of a spine which is in a position of partial flexion, rather than in a fully-erect posture.

Flexion is a wonderful body function when used properly. However, when sustained for long periods of time, flexion can cause inflammatory degeneration or pressure atrophy of the rim of the bodies of the vertebrae, especially at the margins where the stress is accumulated. This increases month-by-month and year-by-year. Flexion also creates compression of all the internal organs in the thoracic and abdominal cavities. Eventually it may produce the ugly symptoms of off-angle head, drooped shoulders and humped back — commonly referred to as slouch-stance.

The lower back muscles are crucial for proper erect posture, and flexion does stretch certain groups of them; but when used excessively, flexion does not strengthen the lower back muscles. When exercising, how many times have you heard, "Stretch forward, bend low?" Have you stopped to reason that many exercises that are supposed to strengthen the abdominal wall and banish the paunch could be harmful? Usually such exercises involve partial flexion from a horizontal or lying position. In doing them, the exerciser lies on his back and raises his legs to various positions; he then raises the trunk and touches the toes. The chief muscles used in these exercises are the psoas, which are the ones that connect the lower back and thigh (femur) bones. The abdominal muscles are not used directly because they are not connected to the thigh, so they cannot be used to change the position of the trunk relative to the thigh. Actually all we are doing is adding to the strain associated with our ordinary movements, and for the older person, this can be dangerous and painful. Frequent repetition of these acts does not encourage good response in postural correction. Knowing this, we can see that the need for antagonistic or balanced postures is vital.

The first basic rule of good posture and adjustment for gravitational effects is this: *Extension must oppose flexion.* We must use both movements to more nearly attain the ideal postural state and the accompanying relief from aches and pains.

Generally orthodox opinion holds that *flexion of the spine* creates:

1. Traction on the dural sac.
2. Upward movement of the spinal nerves.
3. Back and forth dorsal root ganglion migration.
4. Posterior displacement of nucleus palposus. (*)
5. Enlargement of the intervertebral foramina.

41

6. Elongation of the spine.
   When the spine is in total flexion (hyperflexion), it is one-third longer than when the spine is in total extension.
7. Obliteration of the normal lumbar lordosis.
8. Widening of the lumbar and lumbrosacral inter-laminar spaces.
9. Retraction of the nerve roots.

So far we have discussed the three common postures, namely, erect, horizontal and flexed. We now know something about the effects of these postures on the body and the proper way to employ them. We also know that when used exclusively, they can, and usually do, produce adverse effects in our body. In the following chapters we will discuss how to counter the adverse effects of these postures by means of exercises employing three uncommon, oppositional postures, which are Extension, Brachiation, and Inversion.


(*) Latest research questions this.

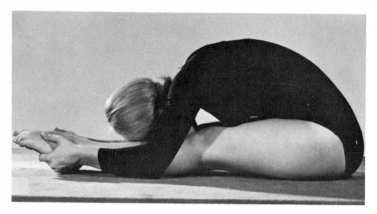

*Fig. 7. — Sitting jackknife*

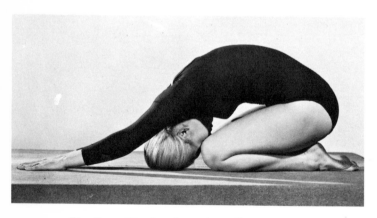

*Fig. 8. — Flexion from kneeling position*

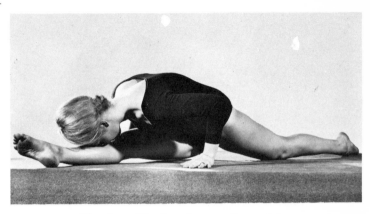

*Fig. 9. — Flexion from split position*

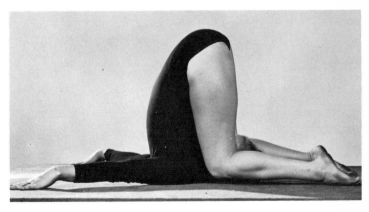

*Fig. 10. — Shoulder jackknife*

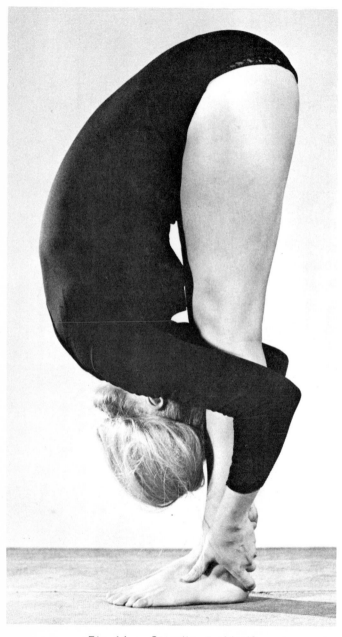

*Fig. 11. — Standing jackknife*

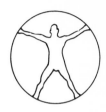

# CHAPTER 10

## *The Extended Posture*

Recall the flexed posture, which is the posture of bending forward. Its differential and oppositional posture is the extended posture.

What is extension, and how is it accomplished? What does it do for your stature and health?

Extension is accomplished simply by bending your body backward. When you lean back and reach for the ceiling to relieve a cramp you are in partial extension. This is only partial because you did not bend backward far enough to extend the bending to the vital areas of thighs and hips.

A word of caution! When you begin extension exercise, approach it gradually since the affected muscles may be stiff or weak from non-use. These muscles may have acquired a major postural debt; reduce this debt slowly until you become accustomed to this exercise.

What will postural extension exercise do for you? First, it helps to correct the basic structural faults produced by excessive partial flexion, as demonstrated by the inability to bend backward freely because of abnormal pelvic tilt and weakened and shortened anterior leg and abdominal muscles. Faults like this must be remedied in order to correct poor posture.

When you bend backward, each segment of the spine rotates on its transverse axis. Shifting direction of pressure on the spinal discs and the vertebrae allows physiological differences of function and effect to safeguard the body's structural health and form.

The first time you bend backward from a kneeling position, you will probably notice that the thigh muscles seem tense and tight. Running, walking, and bending forward have tensed these muscles. Only complete extension can stretch them and allow the pelvis to return to the proper position for spinal balance. Complete extension means bending backward until the body is at least bowed — and more is even better.

What about the muscles on the backside of the thigh and the muscles of the buttocks when in a sitting position? Notice how relaxed and flabby these muscles are. On the other hand, the muscles on the front of the thigh are probably tight. When the muscles in the hamstrings and buttocks become weak they cannot function as postural muscles — as balancers of the pelvis — or as proper antagonists to the shortened, tense extensor muscles located on the front of the thigh.

Complete extension is absolutely necessary to counteract the deleterious effects of sag due to bad posture practice and excessive orthostance. Complete extension practiced with complete flexion aids the spine to become properly positioned for balance. Equally, it strengthens the muscles which do the balancing. It is the equalization of tone produced by these exercises that brings about the balance between the antagonistic muscle groups. This makes the body straight and beautiful. *It can be stated that subluxation anywhere in the body indicates lack of alignment caused by loss of strength between antagonistic muscle groups.*

It has always been a problem for the obstetrician to restore the tone and health of the muscles of the mother following childbirth. Extension exercises aid greatly in solving this problem. Arching backward from the knees fulfills a requirement for adjustment of the pelvic architecture. The anterior (front) torso and leg muscles are usually in poor condition in pregnant women and, for that matter, in most modern women.

It is relatively easy to obtain superb tone in these muscles when the differential exercises of complete extension and complete flexion are performed regularly. These strengthen and balance the pelvic girdle to secure pelvic poise.

Mothers who are trained in gravity guiding exercises return to handstands, arches from the knees, and brachiation within a few days after delivery. These exercises allow gravity to influence the regressing uterus to return to its highest possible anatomical, natural position in the pelvis.

Although these oppositional exercises have shown excellent results, there are some physical educators who continue to advocate avoidance of all extension exercises. Such advocates are afraid that bending backward will weaken the lower back and deepen the inward curve of the spine. However, just the opposite is true. Complete extension will not cause lordosis. *The fact that most of those with lordosis have never practiced extension to any serious degree, and yet have such a prevalent postural fault, gives proof that completely extending the spine does not cause lordosis.*

To straighten, lengthen, and correctively condition the spine is to use the *"rule of all joints,"* that is, *employ maximum mobility. Orthopaedics teaches that complete mobility of a joint is a necessity for joint health and that no joint is excluded. For joint health, every joint must be taken through its full range of motion. The joints of the spine are no exception to this rule of orthopaedics. For the spine to gain its maximum mobility, it must be trained and developed in both complete extension and complete flexion. When the spine is then allowed to relax in the erect posture, the supporting and influencing structures will take the most neutral position between the two extremes of complete extension and complete flexion, thereby minimizing the primary and secondary curves.* To straighten the secondary lumbar curve, one must simultaneously straighten the primary dorsal curve. Complete extension with complete flexion is the answer.

Establishing equilibrium between antagonistic muscle groups will permit the spine to achieve its maximum lengthening and maximum shortening for physiological function. Under correcting and conditioning training, there will be no tendency toward swayback or round shoulders.

No muscle can be strengthened when it is in a condition of constant stretching because its stretch-contracting reflex no longer has the usual response.

Some athletic coaches and physicians employ flexion and more flexion in their attempt to cure swayback and angulation of the hips and lower trunk. Too much partial flexion is already part of the trouble. Under such plan, stretch atrophy will develop in the lumbar region and across the hips (sacroiliacs).

Extension of the spine relaxes the tension of the

meninges, spinal nerves, and cauda equina. This displaces the nucleus palposus anteriorly, minimizes the intervertebral foramina, and shortens the spinal canal. "Long periods of extension tend to realign the vertebrae, relieve pressure on nerves, and heal in proper position." *Today's Health,* June, 1969, p. 6.

Only with complete extension, deliberately practiced as a positional complement of complete flexion, can the muscular components of postural poise become established. These postural components, through muscular isometric tone, will balance and bring about freedom from subluxation and twisted spines.

A beautiful posture depends on joint health, which can be readily attained by almost anyone practicing gravity guidance in a gravitational environment.

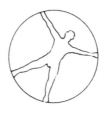

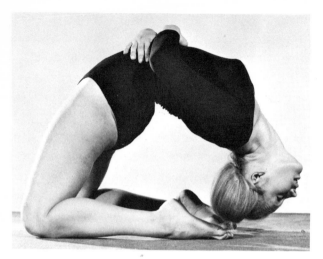

*Fig. 12. — Arch from knees*

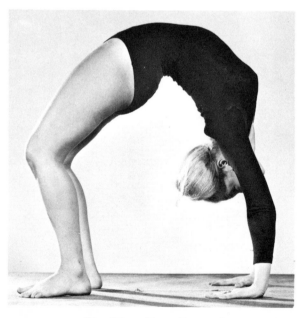

*Fig. 13. — Standing arch*

51

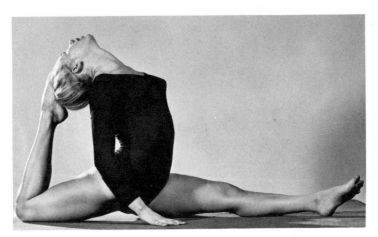

*Fig. 14. — Extension from split position*

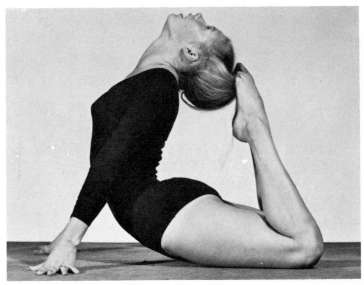

*Fig. 15. — Extension — touch toes to head*

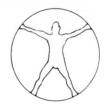

# CHAPTER 11

## *The Brachiated Posture*

**R**ecall the compression effects of the erect posture while sitting or standing. An antagonistic, or oppositional, posture is the brachiated posture (hanging by the arms or legs). Brachiation achieves elongation and decompression of the body.

The dictionary states that *brachial* means "pertaining to the arms;" *brachiate* means "having arms;" and *brachium* means "the upper arm from shoulder to elbow."

To meet our need for a word to denote bearing of the body's weight while suspended by either the arms or the legs, we coined the word *brachiation*. Therefore, in this book, *brachiated posture* will be used to identify one of the six basic differential postures, namely, the posture of hanging by either the arms or the legs.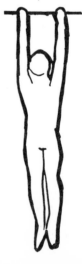

Suspending the body by the arms is a very simple maneuver, yet it is one of the most important therapeutic exercises. Every able-bodied person should do some arm hanging exercises each day, and better yet, do them several times a day. This is an excellent exercise for relief and prevention of common backache.

As something readily accessible to hang from, a round bar, such as a piece of

¾ inch pipe, can be mounted in a doorway.

Even more effective than hanging by the arms is hanging by the legs; this will be discussed in detail in Chapter 12.

One can find records of efforts of practitioners throughout the history of medicine — medieval and modern — who applied the principle of "countering gravity by traction." The aim of such measures was to increase the joint space and joint play in order to relieve pressure points and to straighten and elongate the body.

Today, in hospital and medical offices, one can see all kinds of gadgets and devices used for traction of the body. Unfortunately, most of those advising traction, even those who are teaching stretching exercises, apply it only while the body is in a sitting, standing, or lying position. Traction applied while in these positions negates much of its value.

Also, educational institutions teaching exercise tend to believe that there are no other known postures of the body in which to exercise other than sitting, standing, or lying. The reason for this is that it has generally been considered to be impractical, difficult, or impossible to exercise in any other postures.

Since its weight constantly acts to compress the body, there should be some practical methods available to decompress and elongate it. *There is, to our knowledge, no better way to counteract or neutralize the compressive effect of gravity than to utilize this same gravitational force to effect the opposite, namely, decompression. Suspension of the body from either end offers a great means to apply physiological traction upon the human organism. Brachiation has been largely overlooked as a simple, effective form of traction.* By exercising the body while in extension, inversion, or brachiation, maximum mechanical effect is obtained to pull the tissues and organs headward and to carry the weight away from the sites of usual compression or sag. While hanging by the arms, the body and lower limbs become pro-gravity devices. The stresses in these structures are then exactly opposite from those that exist when the body is supported by the legs in standing.

Hanging by the arms (arm brachiation) is an instinctively natural means of creating traction through the long axis of the body. It may be said to be natural traction since it tones both the pro-gravity and anti-gravity muscles. It is the simplest way to ease strains caused by compression and to lift the weight off the superimposed segments of the body.

*If you are suffering from extreme tension in the back, hang by your arms!* Few exercises are so beneficial in combating both mild and severe cases of back stiffness, such as myositis, fasciitis, and fibrositis. You will be amazed at what such hanging will do. If you have suffered the excruciating pain of bursitis or neuritis, which seem to plague so many these days, brachiation will be a great aid to recovery. Through its application, the erector muscles of the spine become relaxed, and the pressure on the vertebrae and discs of the spinal column is relieved.

In brachiating, the muscles of the shoulders and arms are stretched. Use of the shoulder muscles to brachiate lifts the musculo-skeletal structure of the chest, benefits neck and arm muscles, and expands the chest fully, thus allowing our squashed-down lungs to expand. Also, it tones the abdominal muscles. They are stretched by the upward pull from the chest and intercostal wall, and they automatically tense when the muscles of the back are relaxed. This is reverse-tension reflex of antagonistic muscles. Brachiation is a requirement if you wish to maintain the health of your shoulders and arms.

Rudolph Klapp, a German posture specialist, discovered this reverse-tension reflex interaction some years ago. Recognizing its benefits, he induced it in his patients by having them crawl. (Fig. 18). However, crawling does not replace brachiating as an exercise for the following reasons. In crawling the abdominal muscles contract, and the already over-tense muscles of the frontal thigh shorten and tighten, whereas they stretch when hanging by the arms. Furthermore, crawling does not cause expansion of the chest nor does it develop the shoulder muscles, as does brachiation. Crawling also is not nearly so relaxing to the back and the body as is hanging.

In World War II, it was discovered that a large proportion of our young men had weak arms and torsos. Unfortunately, this condition exists not only in adults but even in our supposedly healthy youngsters.

The Great Architect, in recognizing the importance of musculo-dynamics, gave us an inverted torso cone. This is the shape that gives the human figure the look of eternal youth. The mechanical phenomena of the inverted torso cone is most interesting. When the arms are stretched overhead as high as possible and used to support the entire body weight, the stretching of the torso is a musculo-dynamic act. The torso, suspended from the arms, can be compared with a loaded bucket. The bale is the arms; the upper larger rim of the bucket is the thoracic cage; and the lower rim is the small pelvic ring. Brachiation is the magician who can contour the waist line.

In suspending the body, the mechanism of respiration and the muscles of the abdomen retract the abdominal wall and lift the viscera into the natural elevated position. This strengthening of the abdominal wall is as important as the relaxing of the back. These are reflexively associated. While brachiating, there is no danger of rupture through the inguinal rings, as there may be in the strenuous, upright, foot-supported exercises. To be healthy and vigorous, a person needs a healthy abdominal wall.

The need for postural rehabilitation, contour correction, and common orthopaedic problem prevention makes brachiation a requirement of our way of life. Through brachiation, the weight of the body creates a completely new stress pattern. New physiological opportunity is now offered to the tissues and organs. The very first time you try brachiation by the arms you will feel an exhilaration that somehow satisfies the whole body.

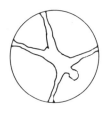

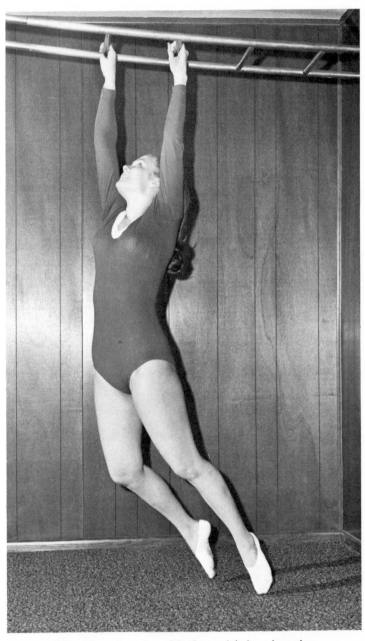

*Fig. 16 — Arm brachiation with legs hanging*

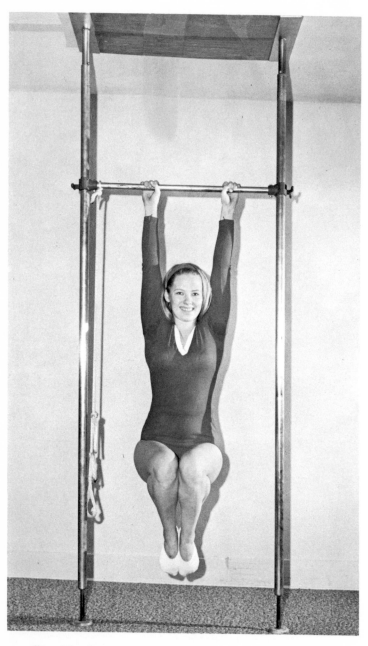

*Fig. 17—Arm brachiation with knees raised and bent*

59

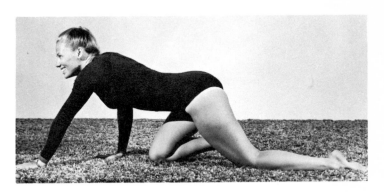

*Fig. 18. — Cross pattern crawling*

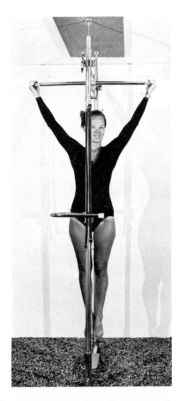

*Fig. 19. — Hanging from toggle bar*

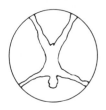

# CHAPTER 12

## *The Inverted Posture*

**R**ecall the *erect* posture, the act of standing or sitting upright. The antagonistic or oppositional posture is the inverted posture. Complete inversion consists of turning the body upside down so that the feet are uppermost and the head is nearest the ground. Lesser degrees of inversion can be attained by lying on an inclined plane with the head downward, such as by lying on an inclined

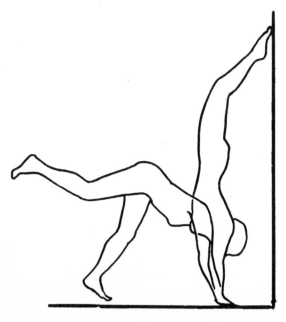

bed, or on a hillside.

Brachiation (hanging) by the lower limbs takes advantage of gravity in a way most profitable to the body. Hanging from the lower limbs, with the body suspended upside down, is a most practical physiological, posture-developing technique. Emphatically, brachiation is diametrically opposite to the compressing posture used when standing on the feet or sitting. In this posture, the force of gravity upon the body is reversed to a maximum degree, thus attaining a much-needed effect of total elongation. In this position all the downward strain produced by erect posture is relieved. The abdomen draws inward and headward instead of sagging footward and outward. The chest is easily expanded, and the diaphragm is pushed and pulled headward. The weakened neck muscles, which in the erect posture fall forward and down to form jowls and double chins, are relieved.

The circulatory system receives extraordinary relief from postural inversion. Inversion relieves the pressure in the lower parts of the body and, at the same time, eases the difficult job of supplying blood to the brain and to the upper parts of the vital organs. Gravity now pulls headward instead of footward, so it is helping the body to support the organs in an elevated manner. Inversion, teamed with gravity, not only helps the muscles and the uncommon tissue warp of the body, but more importantly, it reverses the downward strain on the heart and vascular tree.

Experiments at an Eastern university have revealed that, on an average, the brain operates 7 percent faster and 14 percent more accurately when the body is placed in an inverted, inclined plane.

Scientists at John Hopkins have advanced the hypothesis that the dead air spaces at the top of the lungs are caused by strain resulting from erect posture. Apparently this is caused by failure of blood pressure in the apical capillaries and tissue sagging away from these uppermost spaces when the body is in the erect posture too much.

On the other hand, inversion directs gravity's force in such a way that the dead air spaces in the body are diminished.

For years surgeons have used the semi-inversion posture in the operating room when they are confronted with a patient who is near collapse and in need of circulatory support. In medical vernacular, partial inversion is called Trendelenburg position. Recently, mattress and bedding companies have realized the importance of inversion, not only for normalizing the average person, but also for the seriously ill individual. So they have designed special beds which place the sleeping person in a modified inverted position.

Children will often sleep in an inverted posture, even on a horizontal surface, by assuming a knee-chest position. This naturally relieves the strain of the erect posture. The human fetus is inverted after the period of free flotation, when the fixation time has come for pre-delivery posture. This is in the late stage of uterine development, and for good reasons. In the inverted position the brain has the advantage of gaining the greatest blood supply, thereby assuring advanced brain tissue development by time of birth.

Following birth, an infant is hung upside down by the physician. It is then placed in a crib on an inclined plane so that the head is lower than the body. Subsequently, it should be inverted frequently by the parents; it should also be permitted and encouraged to assume the knees-to-chest posture while napping. An older child should have access to a bar or tree branch from which to swing.

In reducing body weight, a good way to avoid loose jowls flapping over the neck, like that of a turkey gobbler, and to prevent the skin of the cheeks from getting flabby is to reverse the pull of gravity by inverting the body. Also, this method can make an aged person look many years younger.

Assuming an upside-down position will restore sagging internal organs such as the stomach, bowels, uterus, and meningies to their correct positions. It will also be helpful in correcting paralytic scoliosis and inclinatory skeletal defects (rib angle changes, thin discs, and compression wedging of the vertebrae). It can also have beneficial effects in relieving the pressure of a humped back, in flattening a protruding abdomen, in raising and readjusting droopy and protruding hips, and in raising and enlarging a sunken flat chest.

Other effects of inversion that will be noticed immediately are profound relief of the muscles which end at the very bottom of the abdominal wall. This is because the chest expands as the body is inverted, and the diaphragm is then easily raised. Gravity is now pulling with the muscles which lift the chest walls. Even though it is not noticeable, the blood will flow more easily from the legs back to the heart.

If you are constantly tired, reclining with the head lower than the feet on a cum gravity bed (inclined bed) from eight to ten hours will be beneficial. The organs will profit most from inversion practiced regularly every night. Take care to increase the incline of the bed gradually. Avoid symptomatic equilibral disturbances, such as, nausea, full head, headache, etc. Upon feeling any disturbing symptoms, discontinue the practice of this.

Other common troubles that are alleviated when *inversion* is practiced daily are: circulatory ptosis with vascular deterioration (damaged blood vessels, varicose veins, and hemorrhoids); visceroptosis (displaced organs); and structural changes (compression of spine, ribs, chest, back and neck).

Inversion of the body can be accomplished in several ways — some simple, others more difficult. The easiest way to partially invert the body is to lie on an inclined plane with the head downward and the feet upward. Anyone can construct such an inclined plane by simply placing graduated furniture lifts under the footend legs of his bed. In the inverted position, one will feel a rush of blood to the head. The reason for this is that when the body is inverted the pull on the excessively convoluted vessels (blood and lymph), and their contents, is adjusted to physiological advantage. During this change, a more efficient blood and lymph supply reaches the uppermost structures (brain, eyes, ears, etc). The inverted position may at first cause temporary dizziness and nausea in a person not accustomed to the freedom of postural exchange. It may require a few practices to eliminate this. This situation was brought on by the individual's years of sedentary living.

Lack of blood flow to the brain and lower tissues, no doubt plays an important part in geriatric degeneration and premature aging. Why? We know the brain is the center of nerve control and that all movements originate in the brain. When this brain mass lacks a sufficient supply of blood the natural results will be slow body reactions and sluggish mental and physical reflexes — a possible reason for lack of mental alertness and response.

If the vascular capacity of the body is reduced the blood supply to the brain cells is affected as well. Symptoms of vascular changes may become evident in poor memory, inability to make decisions, and in numerous other ways. When these symptoms appear, it is evident from a therapeutic standpoint that postures which alter gravity's effect are vitally needed.

It is impossible to overestimate the importance of maintaining continuous free-flow exchange of blood and other fluids into the extremities of the body. This can be achieved by frequent exchange of the six basic postures.

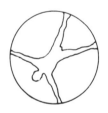

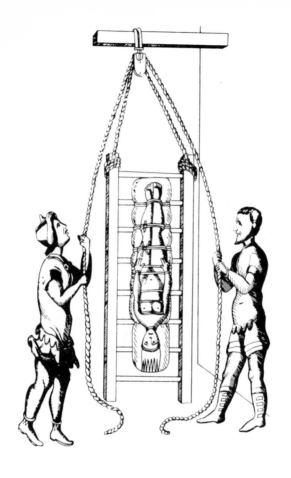

*Fig. 20. — Representation of the ancient mode
of performing succussion.*

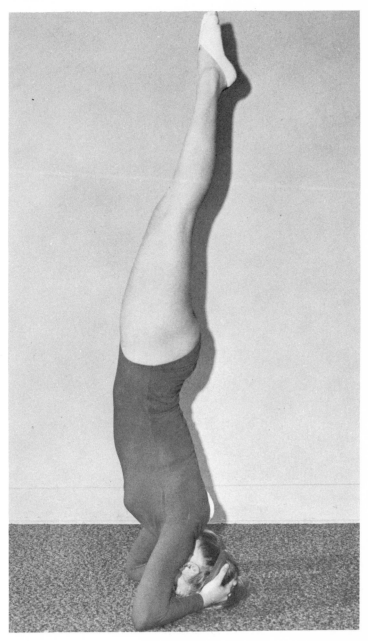

*Fig. 21. — Forearm stand*

68

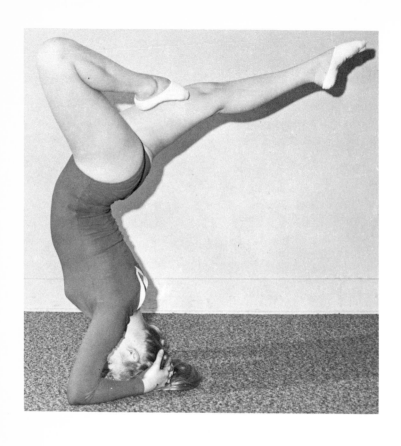

*Fig. 22 — Variation of Forearm stand*

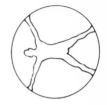

# CHAPTER 13
*Your Physical Fitness Test*

### (Maximum Score - 150)

Now that you know the six basic postures necessary for physical health and what they can do for you, let's find out how physically fit you are. Perhaps you can advance more rapidly in exercising than others because your body is still quite physically adequate. Then again, because you have not used corrective exercises in years, your body may be stiff, weak, and out of condition. Extra care and caution may be required in approaching physical stress of new, but essential, nature. Do not let this discourage you. After all, you will be the one who gets the most benefit from your exercise. Some people engaged in physical-fitness work have set up tests which consist of chinning, pull-ups, running, jumping, throwing a ball, etc. These tests examine the individual through feats which are accomplished almost wholly in the customary common postures. They do not comprehensively test the skill, agility, suppleness, strength, and endurance of the entire body, nor the faculties of equilibrium, proprioceptive perception and reflex.

A true physical fitness test should not only measure your ability in the common postures, but should also measure it in the uncommon postures. For example, a person who can throw a ball does not necessarily have the physical capability to support his body in a headstand against a wall, but a person who can stand on his hands can assuredly throw a ball. Interesting? Who is more physically fit?

Ability to meet all the necessary physiological requirements of the neuro-musculo-skeletal systems, while calling upon the proprioceptive, equilibrial, circulatory exchange mechanism, and reflex response at the same time, determines to a measurable degree the body's fitness.

The test of physical fitness is how well you function in getting in and out of the six basic postures. Speed, endurance, flexibility, strength, agility and spontaneity are all attributes of one who is physically fit. A basic physical fitness test should be applicable to all ages and both sexes. All should be measured against the same standards. We need a standard procedure by which physical comparisons can be made on the basis of over-all physical fitness without regard to chronological age or sex. Only in this way can we obtain a clear picture from our tests of such things as correction required, progress, retrogression, degeneration, and premature old age. Fitness should be related to physiological age rather than to chronological age.

We should think of *physical fitness* as the ability of the body to remain or become healthy, and otherwise live beneficially in its environment. Then it is operating at optimum. In this connection, advantageously adapting the body to the force of gravity is a consideration of paramount importance. Physical fitness is very much dependent upon postural fitness; and postural fitness reaches its ultimate when the body can assume any reasonable position in relationship to gravity. In order to do this, the muscles must be capable of total flexion and extension, and the joints must have full range of motion. It must also be possible to maneuver the body without intolerably disturbing the vascular system, the respiratory mechanism, or the equilibrium.

*Postural efficiency is the foundation of physical fitness.* Understanding the six basic postures, regular practice of them, and the exercises associated with them, are the keys to physical fitness. Therefore, we must clearly recognize the importance of these postures in setting up an adequate physical fitness test.

Do not be discouraged by a poor test score. Most people need help in postural correction, and the exercises described in Chapter 14 of this book are designed to provide the help required. Your possibilities under the *gravity guiding system* are astounding.

### Your Basic Physical Fitness Test

**(1) The** *Erect Posture*
These exercises test the ability of the ankles, knees, hips, and spinal column to function in coordination, and the ability of the legs to lift the body.

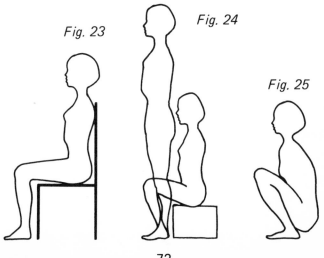

*Fig. 23*

*Fig. 24*

*Fig. 25*

Stand with legs spread and toes turned out. Now, with heels flat on floor, bend knees and squat:

|  | Points |
|---|---|
| To chair seat height (Fig. 23) . . . . . . . . . . . . . . . .1 | |
| To footstool height (Fig. 24). . . . . . . . . . . . . . . .2 | |
| To heel height (full squat) (Fig. 25) . . . . . . . . . . .5 | |
| Total points possible | 8 |

(2) The *Horizontal Posture*

These exercises test the ability to get into and out of the lying posture.

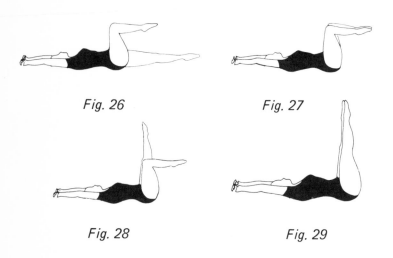

Fig. 26            Fig. 27

Fig. 28            Fig. 29

(A)  Lie on your back with both arms fully extended above the head; then do the following:

|  | Points |
|---|---|
| Raise one bent leg to vertical (Fig. 26) . . . . . . . .1 | |
| Raise both bent legs to vertical (Fig. 27). . . . . . .2 | |
| Raise one straight leg to vertical (Fig. 28) . . . . . .2 | |
| Raise both straight legs to vertical (Fig. 29) . . . .5 | |

(B) Starting from a lying-on-your-back position do
the following situps:

Extend arms above head; then sit up..........1

Place arms at sides; then sit up .............2

Clasp hands behind head; then sit up.........5

Total points possible                        18

(3) The *Flexed Posture*

These exercises test the ability of the body to bend
forward.

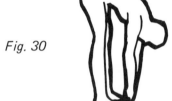

*Fig. 30*

Stand erect; then bend forward with knees straight
(Fig. 30) and do the following:

|  | Points |
|---|---|
| Grasp the knees............................1 |  |
| Grasp the ankles ..........................5 |  |
| Grasp the toes............................10 |  |
| Place forearms behind knees, then touch head to |  |
| knees and hold this position for count of 10....15 |  |
| Total points possible                        31 |  |

(4) The *Extended Posture*

These exercises test the ability to bend backward, and
the flexibility of the anterior (front) muscles of the legs
and body.

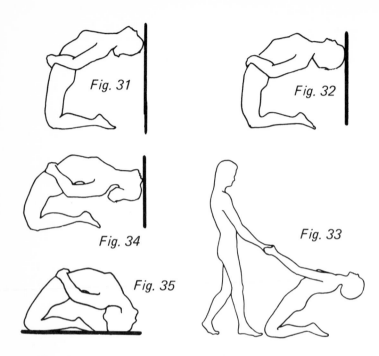

Fig. 31

Fig. 32

Fig. 34

Fig. 33

Fig. 35

Kneel on the floor with your back facing toward a wall. With legs spread comfortably, and with toes of both feet pointing away from your body, clasp your left wrist with your right hand. Bend backward and touch head to wall. (Distances shown below are measured from floor to point where head touches wall).

Points

Touch at 20"; raise up with help . . . . . . . . . . . . . . .1
Touch at 20"; raise up without help (Fig. 31) . . . . .3
Touch at 15"; raise up with help . . . . . . . . . . . . . .2
Touch at 15"; raise up without help (Fig. 32) . . . . .5
Touch at 10"; raise up with help (Fig. 33) . . . . . . .3
Touch at 10"; raise up without help (Fig. 34) . . . . .6
Touch floor; raise up with help . . . . . . . . . . . . . . .10
Touch floor; raise up without help (Fig. 35) . . . . .15
Total points possible         45

(5) The *Brachiated Posture*

These exercises test the usability of the shoulders and arms, and general strength of the torso muscles.

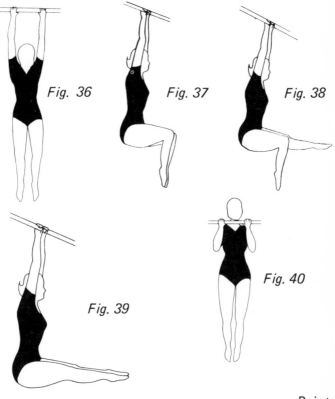

Fig. 36

Fig. 37

Fig. 38

Fig. 39

Fig. 40

Points

From an overhead bar, hang by:

Both arms (Fig. 36). . . . . . . . . . . . . . : . . . . . . . . . . .1

Both arms, with hips turned at right angle to
shoulders, and with both knees bent
(Fig. 37) . . . . . . . . . . . . . . . . . . . . . . . . . . . . . . . .2

Both arms, with hips at right angle to
shoulders, one knee bent, the other leg
straight with toes pointed horizontally
(Fig. 38) . . . . . . . . . . . . . . . . . . . . . . . . . . . . . . . .5

Same as previous exercise except do with
both legs horizontal (Fig. 39) . . . . . . . . . . . . . . .15
Both arms, and chin yourself on the bar
5 times (Fig. 40) . . . . . . . . . . . . . . . . . . . . . . . . .5
Total Points Possible                              28


(6) The *Inverted Posture*

These exercises test the ability to get in to and out of
the upside-down posture.

Do a handstand (stand on your hands) and place your
feet against a wall. Caution: Before attempting this exercise be sure to read the discussion under the heading
"Two-Arm Handstand" in Chapter 14 of this book.

<u>Points</u>

With help (Fig. 41) . . . . . . . . . . . . . . . . . . . . . . . .5
Without help (Fig. 42). . . . . . . . . . . . . . . . . . . . . .15
Total points possible                              20


Maximum possible point total on complete test is 150.

*Fig. 41*

*Fig. 42*

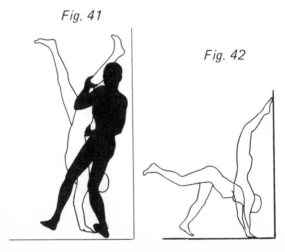

Compare your point total with the following scale:

Outstanding. . . . . . . . . . . . . . . . . . . . . . . . . . . .150
Excellent. . . . . . . . . . . . . . . . . . . . . . . . . . . . .135
Good (minimum physiological economy) . . . . . .100
Fair. . . . . . . . . . . . . . . . . . . . . . . . . . . . . . . . .80
Poor . . . . . . . . . . . . . . . . . . . . . . . . . . . . . . . .50

All of the movements in the foregoing test are physically very elementary. Thus, *the test is basic for people of all ages.* A low score normally reflects the effects of sedentary or improper living and, conversely, demonstrates the need for disciplined, active living. Anyone scoring 80 or less on this test has lost some functional economy and is well along the road to premature old age.

Since you have come this far in this book, you now have some idea of body functions and the essentiality of exercises which properly serve your body's physiological needs. It is urged that you challenge yourself to build your score to 150; this is truly within the capability of all but a few.

In the following chapters we will describe exercises which can assist you to improve your health and beauty — the degree of improvement depends on your willingness to use them.

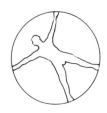

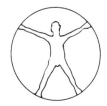

# CHAPTER 14

## Corrective Exercises Which Meet Your Body's Physiological Needs

In this chapter we will endeavor to describe exercises which will promote holistic physical fitness and health, lead to correction of conditions produced by physical stress, and help *to develop and maintain a pain-free back.*

All motion is classified as exercise, but it does not necessarily follow that all such exercise is good or corrective. To truly promote physical fitness, exercise must be discriminate, that is, to be beneficial and effective, exercises must be principled to anatomical needs, rather than selected at random. *The value of motion in corrective exercise depends upon the posture the body is in at the time the exercise is performed.*

The importance of this is evident when we consider the magnificent lattice construction of the body's tissues. The matrix of bone is laid in direct opposition to the lines of stress. The fibrils of intervertebral discs are laid horizontal to the lines of stress. There is an amazingly large variety of joint design to meet the many different requirements in the different parts of the body; also the disposition of the plates of spongy substance of cartilage is in line with the pressures produced by tension.

These, and many more, anatomical and physiological factors determine what forms exercises should take to make them correctional and beneficial.

We have learned that use of the 3 common postures in our every day living — erect, partially flexed and horizontal — tends to develop serious stresses and maladies in our body, caused by the incessant pull of gravity. The following exercises are designed to *employ this same gravity* to counter, relieve, and correct such problems through postural exchange, that is, through exercise in the uncommon postures: extended, brachiated, and inverted.

*Inversion Exercises*

The term Inversion Exercises will be used herein to describe exercises which are performed while the body is in an inverted position, that is, with the head downward and rump upward.

*Forearm Stand - (Figs. 43 and 44)*

Method: Kneel on a carpeted floor. Bend forward, and place top of head on floor. Clasp fingers of the two hands together and place hands behind and against the head. Press forearms firmly to floor with elbows comfortably spaced. Now, by one leg or by both, push the rump up over the head. You are now in an "inverted poodle stand." When you can also raise the legs straight up, you will be in a forearm stand.

*Two-Arm Handstand - (Figs. 46 and 47)*

The two-arm handstand exercise has great therapeutic value; it is among the most beneficial of exercises. But mere mention of it to the uninitiated usually elicits the remark, "Oh! I could never, never stand on my hands." At our institution we teach ambulatory people of all ages to stand on their hands — even grandparents.

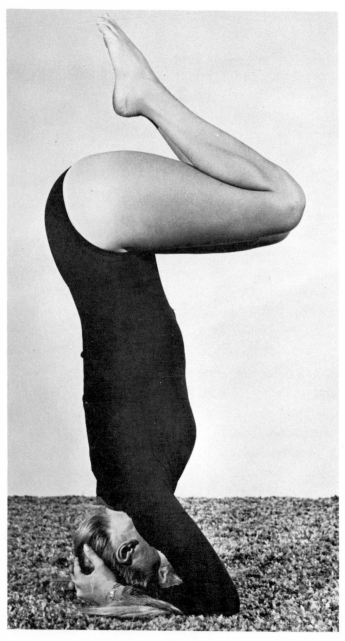

*Fig. 43 — Poodle stand*

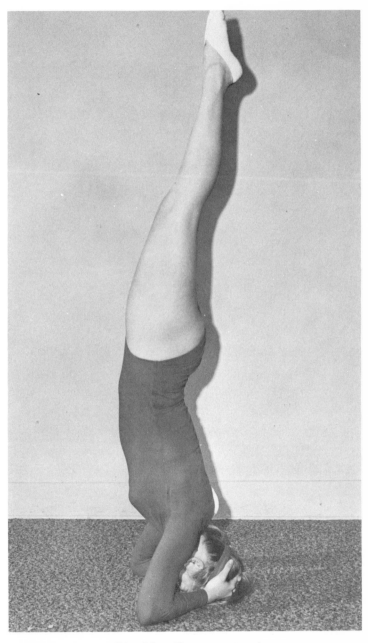

*Fig. 44 — Forearm stand*

Some of our people like to use a Handstand Trainer, as shown in Figs. 47 to 49. Some use this only while learning; others prefer to continue to use it indefinitely. However, the handstand can be readily learned without such device; but an assistant is then necessary while learning. *Caution:* While learning this exercise, always have an able bodied aid assist you until you have become self-sufficient in doing it. The aid should stand at your right side, as shown in Fig. 45, and remain there throughout the exercise. He should help you to get your feet up and to get them back down, and he should particularly prevent you from falling while you are in the inverted position.

Method: Stand, facing a sturdy wall. Now bend forward and place the palms of both hands on the floor, 16 to 24 inches from the wall. Extend straight right leg behind you with tip of foot touching floor. Bend left knee. Now push off by straightening the left knee and simultaneously swinging the straight right leg up and over the head until the sole of its foot meets the wall. As the right leg swings up, the left leg follows until the sole of its foot also meets the wall. You are now in a two-arm handstand. Hold this position as long as comfortable. To come down, start the left leg down first and follow with the right leg; the object is to land on the left foot first. Do not bring both feet down together. Now rest, and then repeat this procedure 5 to 10 times.

If you are in poor condition — weak, stiff, suffering from arthritis — you may continuously need the help of an assistant to do this exercise. Nevertheless, try to do it as the benefits are well worth the effort.

In doing the handstand with the feet against a wall, you will be obtaining the primary and major benefits of this exercise. However, you may want to try some advancements in this skill. Having advanced to this point, it will be relatively easy to learn the free handstand in which you balance on the hands without touching the feet to the wall. A following logical advancement from here is to learn to walk on the hands; you will be very proud of yourself when you can hand walk forward, and even more proud if you can also hand walk backward.

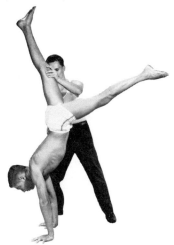

*Fig. 45. — Two-arm handstand with assistance*

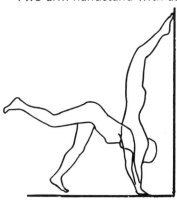

*Fig. 46. — Two-arm handstand against a wall without assistance*

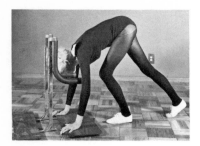

*Fig. 47*

*Fig. 48*

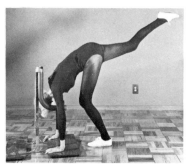

*Fig. 49*

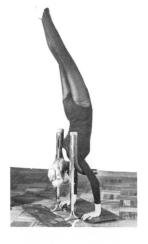

*Three views showing use of Handstand Trainer. Fig. 47, starting position. Fig. 48, pushing with left leg and swinging right leg upward. Fig. 49, in handstand position.*

*Sitting Jackknife - (Flexion in a sitting position) - (Fig. 50)*

Method: While sitting on the floor, bend forward as far as possible with the knees kept straight. Hold this position for a count of 10. Return to the beginning position. Try to repeat this procedure 10 times.

Purpose: To lessen lumbar curvature; to widen the lumbar and lumbosacral interlaminar spaces; and to cause retraction of the spinal nerve roots.

Note: Postural exchange results in physiological change. Muscles tone, loosen, and develop; capsular and fascial structures become free, ligaments and tendons lengthen; adhesions, osteoporosis, and soft tissue fibrosis tend to be eliminated.

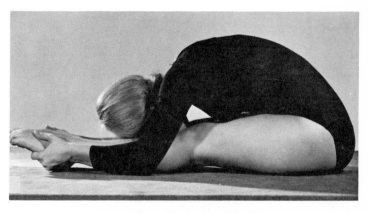

*Fig. 50. — Sitting jackknife*

*Leg Squat (Fig. 51)*

Stand with feet spread comfortably, toes pointing slightly outward, and back erect. Place your hands on your hips; or preferably, clasp hands together and place them behind your head. Keep heels on floor. Now alternately squat and stand in continuous motion. During any one exercise, strive to do this 60 to 100 times in sets of 20.

When first learning this exercise, squat to chair seat height. As your body becomes trained, progressively lower the rump further until it touches the heels; you will then be doing "deep knee bends".

Comment: This exercise promotes blood circulation, tones and strengthens the muscles of the legs; and conditions the ankles, knees, and hip joints. It is also an excellent back conditioner.

*Fig. 51.*
*Leg squat*

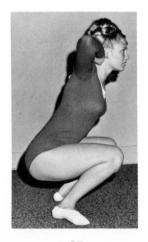

*Arch From Knees (Extension in kneeling position)*
*(Fig. 52)*

Method: Kneel on a padded floor, with legs spread comfortably and with the toes of both feet pointing away from your body. Clasp either wrist with your other hand. Now bend backwards as far as possible or until your head touches a wall or padded chair seat. Hold this position for a count of 10. Return to the beginning position. Try to repeat this procedure 10 times.

In progressive exercises, bend your back further until you can finally touch your head to the floor and return to the beginning kneeling position without assistance of hands.

Purpose: To mobilize the joints in extension and aid development of spinal health.

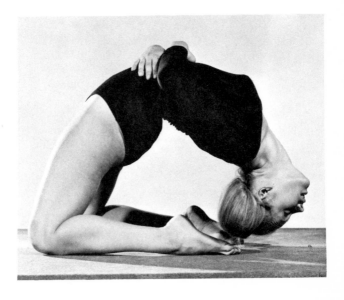

*Fig. 52. — Arch from knees*

*Standing Jackknife (Flexion in standing position)*
*(Fig. 53)*

Method: Stand erect. Now with knees straight (not bent) bend forward at the waist and try to touch fingers, or palms of hands, to the floor. Hold this position for a count of 10. Return to starting position. Rest. Then repeat procedure 10 times.

In progressive exercises increase the amount of forward bending until you can touch the forehead to the knees.

Purpose: To attain total mobility.

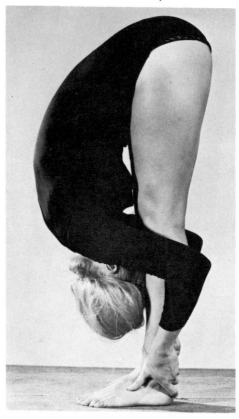

*Fig. 53. — Standing jackknife*

*Shoulder Jackknife — (Fig. 54)*

Method: Lie on back with legs fully extended and with arms fully extended and placed alongside the thighs. With arms remaining in place on floor, swing your legs over your head, keeping legs straight, and try to touch floor with toes. (After you can do this, bend knees and touch knees to floor). Hold this position as long as comfortable, or as long as desired. Return to starting position. Rest. Then repeat this procedure as desired.

Comment: Motion is not physiological exercise unless the joints are put through their full range of motion.

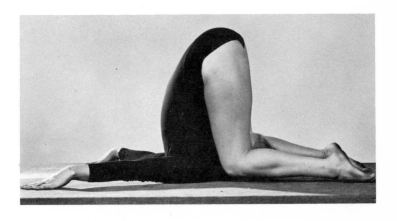

*Fig. 54. — Shoulder jackknife*

*Standing Arch (Extension in a Standing Position)*
*(Fig. 55)*

Method: With feet spaced to provide a firm stance, stand approximately 3 feet from a wall. Face away from wall and raise both hands above head. Now arch backward until your hands touch the wall. Return to beginning position. Try to repeat this procedure 10 times. In progressive exercises, increase the amount of arch until you can eventually touch your hands to the floor.

Purpose: To realign the vertebrae; relieve pressure on nerves; permit antepulsion of the discs; and to attain total mobility of the spine and pelvis.

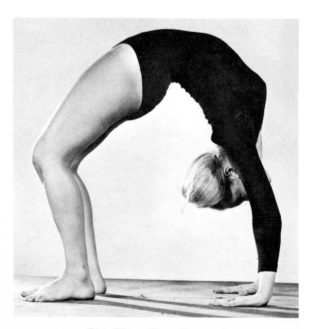

*Fig. 55. — Standing arch*

*Back Stretch (Extension) - (Fig. 56)*

Method: Securely mount a horizontal bar (such as a piece of ¾ inch pipe) about 40 inches above the floor — adjust height to suit. Kneel, grasp bar with both hands with palms facing away from you, and with elbows bent slightly. Next, lean forward as far as possible, thus arching the back. Bend neck backward. Now sway the back 10 times. Then return to beginning position. Rest. Then repeat this procedure 10 times. To increase amount of back arch, move position of knees forward.

An added variation: While back is arched, lift both feet and try to touch them to back of head.

Purpose: To stretch and lengthen the anterior (front) muscles.

Comment: Multiple postures lead to permanent correction of subluxation. To be free of subluxation, the spine requires equalized stress.

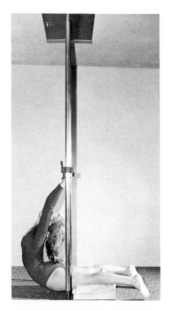

*Fig. 56. — Back stretch*

*Press Up Arch (Extension) - (Fig. 57)*

Method: Lie on your back on a rug (a rug is required for traction). Bend knees and pull feet close to buttocks with feet about 15 inches apart. Bend elbows and place hands on floor alongside of your ears, with fingers pointing toward heels. Now push body up into a backward arch and hold this position for a count of 10. Return to beginning position. Rest. Then repeat procedure 10 times.

Purpose: To strengthen the extensor muscles, and lengthen the flexor muscles.

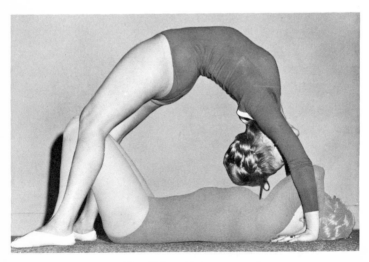

*Fig. 57. — Press up arch*

*Hanging by the Arms (Arm Brachiation) - (Fig. 58)*

This exercise consists of hanging by the two arms from an overhead bar (or other suitable object) with the palms of the hands facing away from you. Preferably, the height of the bar should be adjustable so that it can be raised until the feet just clear the floor when hanging fully suspended. Hang until you feel stress. Do this by count, and in progressive exercises increase the count. If you must hang with the knees bent and feet touching the floor, do so, since this is still very beneficial.

Sufficiently agile persons can do additional challenging exercises when hanging from an overhead bar by the arms, such as: draw-over, draw-around, planch, chin, "skin the cat", toggle, etc.

Note: Hanging or swinging while suspended in this manner is a very simple but highly beneficial, exercise. Every ablebodied person should do it several times daily. A few minutes a day spent on this exercise will pay big dividends in relief of stress.

Purpose: In this elongated posture, the arm and shoulder joints and the vertebral joints are relieved of fixations, compression, and impaction, thus counteracting adverse effects incurred during long hours of standing and/or sitting.

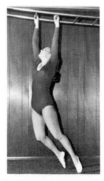

*Fig. 58. — Hanging by the arms*

*Partial Inversion While Sleeping or Resting (Fig. 59)*

Method: Place a disk — 1 inch thick — under each of the foot-end feet of your bed so as to position your feet higher than your head; leave the disks in place. Add a disk at intervals of one month so as to gradually accustom yourself to the change in position. Continue until the foot-end of the bed has been raised 6 to 10 inches.

Note: Disks can be homemade, as from wood, or can be obtained commercially.

Comment: This provides rest at its best. The cumulative effects of gravity, while in the erect position throughout the day, will be countered by sleeping in an inclined position with the head lower than the feet.

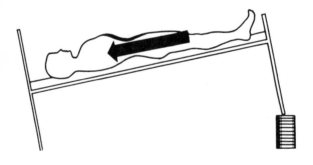

*Fig. 59. — Resting in an inclined bed*
*with head lower than feet*

*Toggle Bar Exercise (Figs. 60 and 61)*

Method: Grip the toggle bar near its ends. With the body suspended, pull down on one end of the bar and simultaneously push up on the other end as far as possible. Now alternately raise and lower the two ends of the bar in a slow, continuous motion.

Purpose: To bring the shoulders into overhead stressful use. The alternate side-to-side traction elevates and develops the rib cage. Torquing of the torso tends to straighten the lateral (scoliosis) weight-bearing curvatures of the spine. In this exercise weight bearing is away from the joint spaces. The alternate push and pull of the arms shifts stress throughout the lateral spinal supports.

Comment: To have full, healthy joint play, the joint must be exercised in compression and separation. Joint physiology requires "joint milking", that is, alternate pressure on and off of the joint.

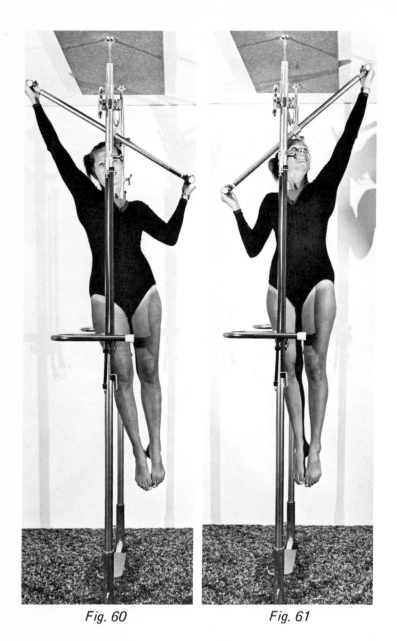

Fig. 60                    Fig. 61

*These views show the two alternate positions of the toggle bar exercise.*

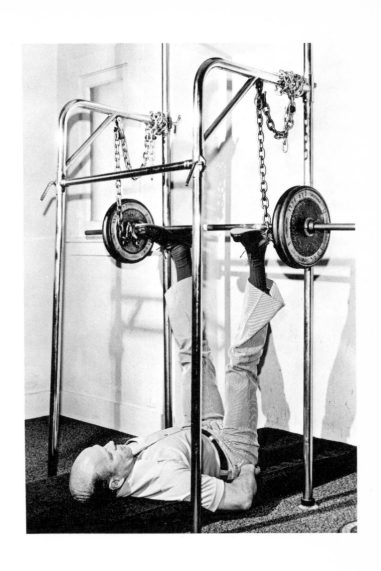

*Fig. 62. — Sole Press exercise*

*Sole Press Exercise (Fig. 62)*

This exercise consists of lifting barbell weights with the legs while lying on your back on the floor. A standard barbell assembly is employed but adapted to the required use.

The bar of the barbell is suspended from a metal frame by a pair of metal chains which are secured to the bar about 18 inches from each end of the bar. Weights of any desired amount are slipped onto the two ends of the bar and secured in place by the conventional bar clamping collars. The effective length of the chains should be readily adjustable at their upper ends so as to suit the need of each individual. Thus the barbell assembly is in free floating suspension, that is, it can move in any direction. within the constraint of the chains; *this is a most important factor in this exercise.*

The bar is pushed upward with the soles of the feet; hence the name *Sole Press* exercise. The bar should contact the soles of the shoes at the arches. Shoes with thick soles, preferably leather, should be worn to pad the feet, and the shoes must have heels to aid in keeping the bar from rolling off the soles.

The preparatory procedure is as follows. Lie on your back on a padded surface on the floor with your hips directly beneath the hanging barbell. Clasp both hands behind your head, and place the soles of your shoes up against the hanging bar. The height of the bar should be such that the knees are fully bent when the soles touch the bar; if it is not, adjust the height accordingly. Move the position of the body footward or headward as required in order to balance the weighted bar on your shoes as you raise and lower it with your legs.

The exercise procedure is as follows. Push the barbell up by straightening the knees until the legs are straight and rigid. Then hold this position for a few seconds. You are now both supporting and balancing the barbell with your legs and feet. Now lower the barbell about a third of the way .by bending the knees, and then immediately raise it back up by straightening the knees. Again hold it in this position for a few seconds before again lowering it. Continue this sequence in a rhythmic manner, accompanied by count of number of times, until you tire. Then remove your feet from the bar and stretch out and rest. Repeat this procedure as often as desired.

Begin with a small amount of weight on the bar, an amount which you can handle comfortably, such as two 5 pound or two 10 pound weights. It generally requires some practice to learn to keep the barbell balanced on the feet, but it is the muscular effort and muscular coordination required to maintain this balance which provides pronounced therapeutic benefits. After you have learned the technique, gradually add weights. The goal of any well conditioned person should be to sole press an amount of weight equal to twice the weight of his body, and to do this 100 to 150 times in sets of 25 to 50. We have had persons of average build who could sole press 700 pounds, but for normal exercising, the emphasis should not be on maximum amount of weight but rather on the number of times a reasonable amount of weight can be lifted.

In doing this exercise you are exercising the strongest muscles of the body in isolation (they are not teamed with the weaker muscles of the back), and thus exerting these great muscles to their maximum. The combination of weight lifting and weight balancing with the legs is highly beneficial to restoration of lost mobility of the legs, knees, hips and, importantly, the pelvis and back. All are compelled to respond and to do so in close coordination with each other. Additionally, marked advantages are provided to those soft tissues which are often responsible for the torments of sciatica and sacroiliac conditions. In brief, this exercise is highly valuable for conditioning and strengthening the muscles of the legs and back, restoring coordination of these muscles, and correcting lower back problems.

The equipment used in this exercise must be properly designed and constructed to assure that the weight loaded bar will not accidentally fall on the exerciser. Equipment similar to that shown in Fig. 62 is commercially available, either as a separate unit, or as an accessory of the GRAVITY GUIDER (Fig. 69).

### Hanging-Inverted Exercises

Hanging-inverted exercises are performed while hanging by the legs. One of the great needs of the body is to be stretched and elongated (traction) so as to counteract the compressive effects of sitting and standing. An excellent way to fulfill this need is to exercise while hanging by the legs. In this position, the pull of gravity on the body is in the headward direction. A word of caution: When first starting, do not hang upside down longer than is comfortable. During the first few times of hanging upside down, some people experience some nausea or dizziness, but upon returning to the upright position, such symptoms disappear in a few minutes. After becoming accustomed to hanging upside down and after doing it a few times, most people enjoy its benefits more and more.

Probably the major deterrent, in the past, to exercising while hanging inverted has been the lack of suit-

able, safe, comfortable means to support the legs. To fulfill such requirements, INVERSION BOOTS (*) were developed. A pair of these boots is shown in Fig. 63. The boots fit around the ankles. Essentially, each boot consists of two sturdily constructed metal half-cylinders. These are joined on one side by a hinge which allows the boot to be opened and then closed around the ankle; on the other side is a draw-pull latch for quickly securing the boot. Attached to each boot is a U-shaped hook for hooking over a round bar. The inside of the boot is lined with a soft, resilient material to provide comfort. Through use of padding (not part of the boot), a single size boot will accommodate all persons except very young children.
(*) Patented; commercially available.

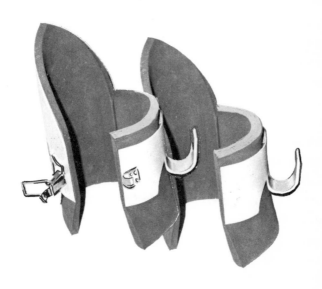

*Fig. 63. — INVERSION BOOTS*

Most of the following described inverted exercises can be performed by hanging from a simple, round bar of adequate strength, such as a ¾ inch pipe. Such bar can be installed in a doorway (not for very tall people), or other suitable place, but should be high enough so the body can hang fully suspended.

An agile person can use the draw-up technique to hook his Inversion Boots onto the overhead bar. This consists of starting from a full arm hang and then drawing the legs up and hooking the boots onto the bar. But only the agile can do this. So we need other methods whereby practically anyone can hang upside down by his feet. One such method is the following described "stirrup" technique.

Tie a non-slipping loop in one end of a strong rope, with the loop made large enough to easily slip over the toe end of your shoe. Then tie the other end of the rope to the overhead horizontal bar. Normally, the loop should hang about 4 feet above the floor, but adjust the rope length to suit.

The procedure for using the stirrup is shown in Figs. 64 to 68 and is as follows: Place either foot in the loop (stirrup) by guiding the loop onto the foot with one hand while supporting your balance with the other hand. Now grab the overhead bar with both hands. Next, step on the foot in the loop (looped foot) and simultaneously pull with the arms until you get the Inversion Boot of the other leg hooked onto the overhead bar. Then hook the "looped foot" onto the bar. (Do not remove the loop). Now let yourself down (Fig. 67) and hang inverted. Then do your exercises.

To get down, reverse the procedure. Start by bending upward from the waist. If you can bend up and reach the overhead bar with your hands, fine; but if you cannot do this, then pull yourself up by grabbing the dangling rope and pulling yourself up until you can firmly grab the overhead bar with both hands. Next, make certain to unhook the "looped foot" first. Now, while supporting your weight by the "looped foot" in the stirrup and by your two hands clasped to the overhead bar, unhook the other foot and bring it to the floor. Then remove the loop in the same manner as when putting it on.

There are a great many people for whom hanging inverted exercises are highly beneficial, but who in the past were unable to get into a hanging-inverted position by themselves, or even with help, because they were disabled, weak, or advanced in age. To enable such people to easily and comfortably get into a hanging inverted position, the following described equipment was developed.

In the hanging-inverted exercises described herein and shown in the accompanying illustrations, a GRAVITY GUIDER (*) is employed. This is a very versatile, multi-function exercising device on which many exercises can be performed. It occupies relatively small space, and can be erected in any ordinary sized room without need for extra mounting accessories. The complete unit is shown in Fig. 69.

One of the components of this unit is the Oscillation Bed, shown being used in Figs. 75 to 78. By means of this Oscillation Bed, almost anyone of any age can, by oneself, easily get into a completely inverted position or into any desired degree of partial inversion. By simply moving the outstretched arms overhead, you can rotate your
(*) Patented; commercially available.

104

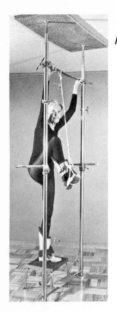

Fig. 64

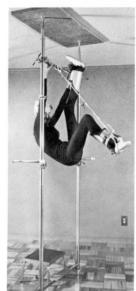

Fig. 65

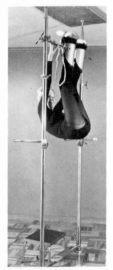

Fig. 66

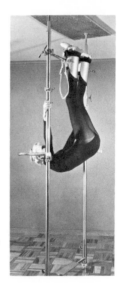

Fig. 67

Figs. 64 through 68 show stirrup technique being used to get suspended in a completely inverted position — by a 79 year young lady.

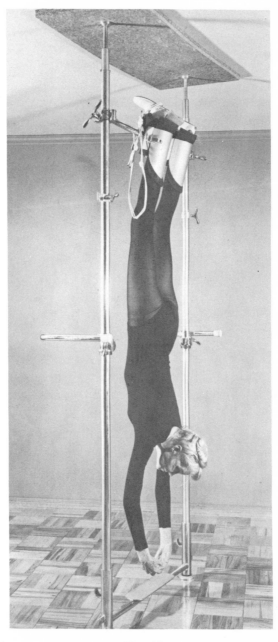

*Fig. 68*

106

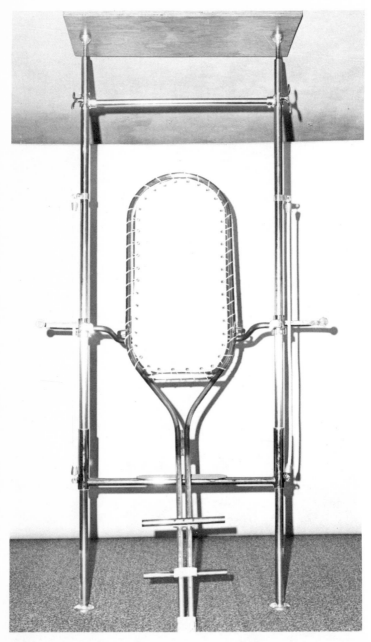

Fig. 69. — *GRAVITY GUIDER; complete unit is shown*

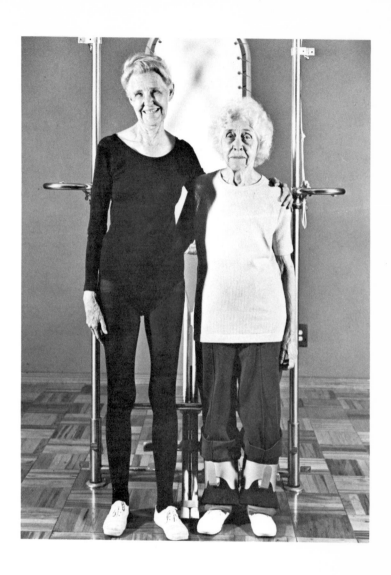

Fig. 70. — *Betty, age 79 (left) and Alice, age 86. Four years before this photo was taken, Alice suffered multiple fractures of the pelvis and fracture of several vertebrae, sustained in an accident. These ladies will be recognized in other photos included herein.*

body to the completely inverted position and remain in this position as long as desired. To return to the upright position, the outstretched arms are moved to the thighs.

The procedure for mounting the Oscillation Bed is shown in Figs. 71 to 74, and is as follows: After putting on the Inversion Boots, stand with your back to the Oscillation Bed (Fig. 71), while holding to the support frame. Next hook the boot of the left foot to the top foot bar from underneath (Fig. 73) and slide the foot to the center support of the bed. Then, in like manner, hook the right foot to the top footbar from underneath. Both feet are now hooked to the top footbar, while standing on the bottom footbar. Thus, the feet are securely fastened to the bed; when in the upright position, the body weight is supported by the bottom footbar, and when in the inverted position, it is supported by the boots hooked to the top footbar (Fig. 74).

The position of the footbars is adjustable to accomodate different size people.

### Full Body Oscillation (Figs. 75 to 78)

The Oscillation Bed gets its name from one of its main functions, namely, that it is used to oscillate the body. By arm movement only, anyone can move his body to any desired position from head up to feet up, or any position in between. With a little practice, he will quickly learn to oscillate his body from head up to feet up, and then reverse this, in a smooth, rhythmic oscillation. This produces an exhilarating feeling. Emphasis is on doing this rhythmically. Advanced age people have no difficulty doing this; in fact, for many aged persons, this is their prime exercise.

Some of the marked physiological benefits (called

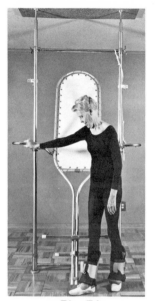

Fig. 71

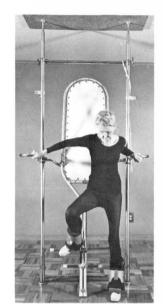

Fig. 72

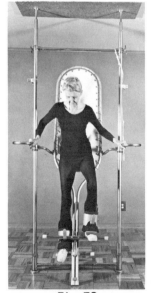

Fig. 73

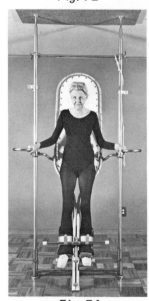

Fig. 74

*Views showing the procedure of mounting the Oscillation Bed*

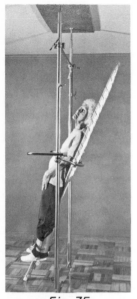

Fig. 75

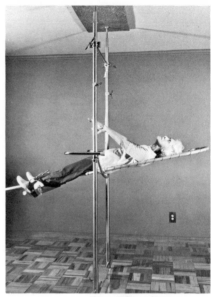

Fig. 76

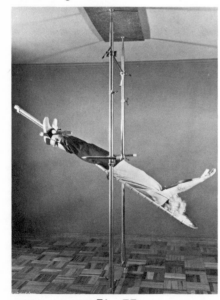

Fig. 77

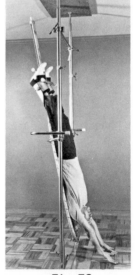

Fig. 78

*Views showing Alice oscillating on the Oscillation Bed;*
*one half of the oscillation cycle is shown*

"dumping effects") to be obtained from this rhythmic postural exchange are: mechanical displacement of fluids, tissues and organs; rhythmic alteration of stress, spinal fluid wash, lymphatic pump effect, and change in hydrodynamics of the vascular circulatory tree. Hundreds of cubic centimeters of blood flow into and out of various parts of the body. The position of the heart shifts, and the density of the lung tissues increases and decreases as the intrathoracic blood volume increases and decreases.

Essentially, this exercise consists of changing the position of the body relative to the pull of gravity in a predetermined, controlled manner so as to employ gravity to produce many highly beneficial therapeutic effects.

Following are descriptions and illustrations of some hanging-inverted exercises:

## Body Rotation (Fig. 79 and 80)

Place hands behind neck and pull elbows close together so arms will not hit the uprights of the exercising unit as the body is rotated. Alternately turn the body, first one way and then the other way, and continue as desired. This exercise will separate the joints and pull various organs headward, thus relieving the body of many symptoms of compression.

## Full Body Swing (Fig. 81)

Swing the extended arms and simultaneously bend the back in the same direction; this will cause the body, suspended on the boot hooks, to swing back and forth like a pendulum. You will be able to swing through a large arc. You should feel a pleasant, rippling feeling along the entire length of the spine.

## Inverted Set-Up (Fig. 82)

Try to touch forehead to knees and hold position for a count of 10. This is an advanced, challenging exercise.

## Inverted Squat (Fig. 83)

Pull up with the legs, and push up with the arms. Hold position for a count of 10. Pull up and let down in an alternating sequence as often as desired.

## Inverted Extension-Flexion Combination (Fig. 84 and 85)

In this lower limb brachiation exercise, you do back-bends. Grip the upright bars at waist height, and push out to arms length. With arms and legs held straight, elevate the rump as high as possible; then let the rump drop down and let the back sag as much as possible. Repeat as desired.

## Weight Lifting in the Inverted Position (Figs. 86 and 87)

The figure shows a young lady being lifted. However, barbell weights, in any desired amount of weight, may be substituted by placing them on the Assist Mechanism on which the young lady is standing.

Figs. 88 to 99 illustrate additional exercises which can be performed without assistance. Figs. 100 to 106 illustrate some of many exercises which can be performed with the aid of an assistant. Imagination can conceive many more.

Obviously, inversion lends itself well to professional therapy, but that is not within the scope of this book. If you have chronic physical problems, by all means see your doctor, first.

The Best of Health to You!

R. Manatt Martin, M.D.
Pasadena, Calif.

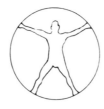

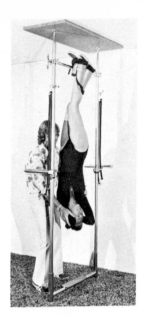

*Fig. 79*

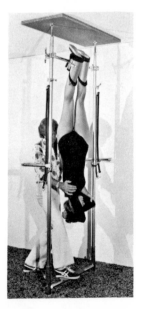

*Fig. 80*

*Figs. 79 and 80 show body rotation — first one way
then the reverse way*

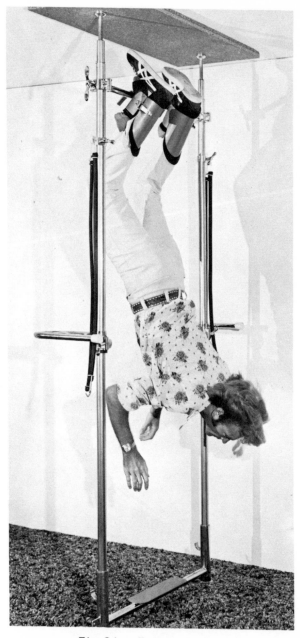

*Fig. 81 — Full body swing*

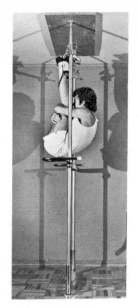

*Fig. 82. — Inverted set-up*

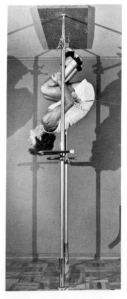

*Fig. 83. — Inverted squat*

117

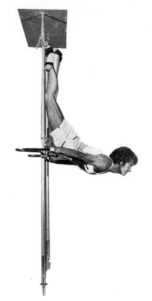

*Fig. 84. — Inverted extension*

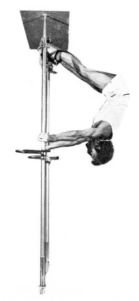

*Fig. 85. — Inverted flexion*

118

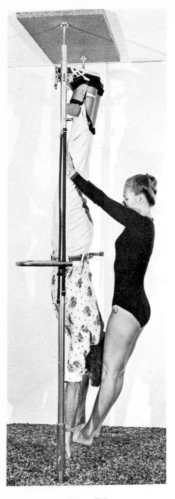

Fig. 86

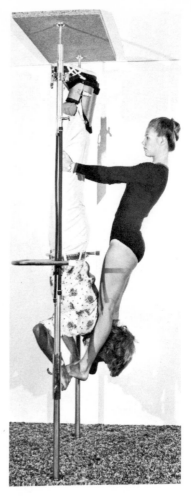

Fig. 87

*Weight lifting in the inverted position —*
*to aid elongation and decompression*

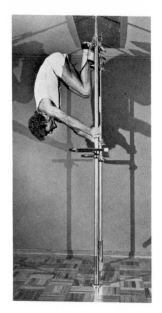

Fig. 88. — *Inverted squat with aid of arms*

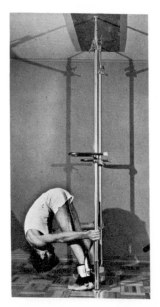

Fig. 89. — *Augmented standing jackknife*

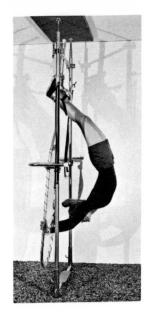

*Fig. 90. — Inverted arch while on Oscillation Bed*

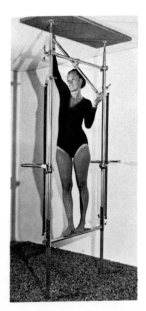

*Fig. 91. — Toggle exercise with aid of Assist Mechanism*

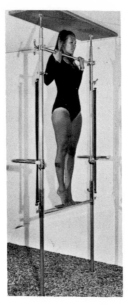

*Fig. 92. — Chinning with aid of Assist Mechanism*

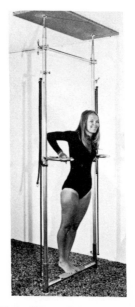

*Fig. 93. — Parallel dips with aid of Assist Mechanism*

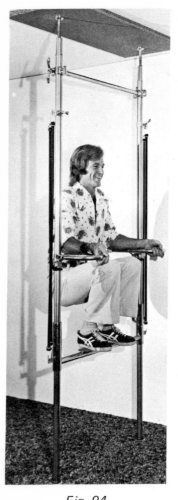

Fig. 94

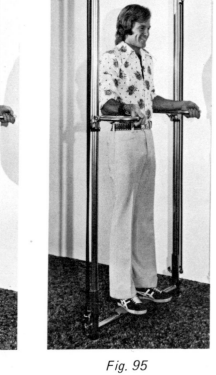

Fig. 95

*Squat with aid of Assist Mechanism*

123

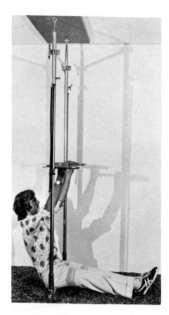

*Fig. 96*

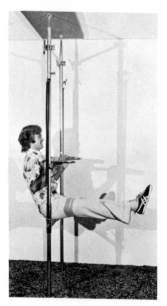

*Fig. 97*

*Handicapped chinning from parallel bars
with aid of Assist Mechanism*

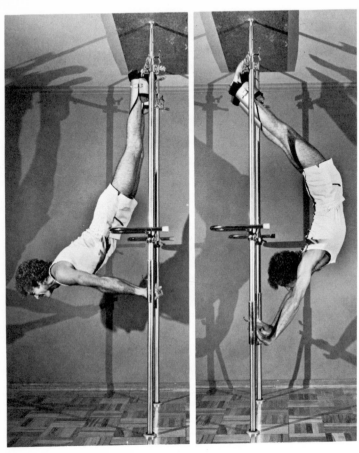

Fig. 98                              Fig. 99

*Draw-up — and — swing through, performed in repetitive*
*sequence*

125

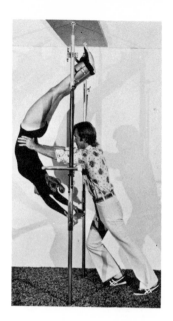

*Fig. 100. — Manipulated backpress*

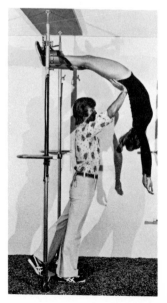

*Fig. 101. — Manipulated extension*

*Fig. 102*

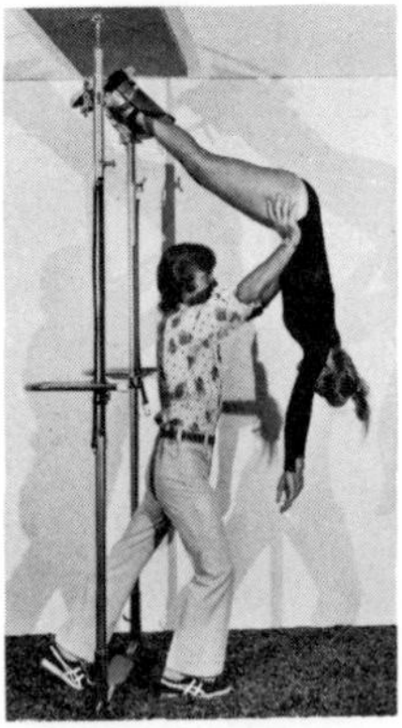

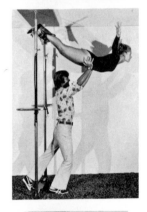

*Fig. 103*

*Fig. 104*

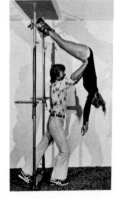

*Front lever (Fig. 102) to Swan (Fig. 103) to Front lever (Fig. 104) performed in repetitive sequence*

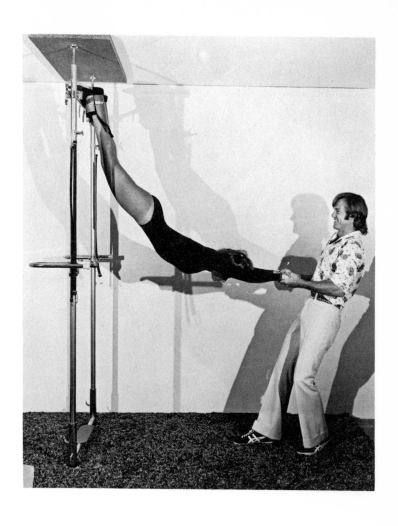

*Fig. 105. — Forced elongation in extension*

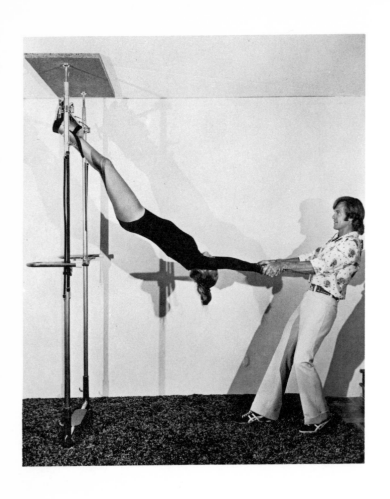

*Fig. 106. — Forced elongation in flexion*

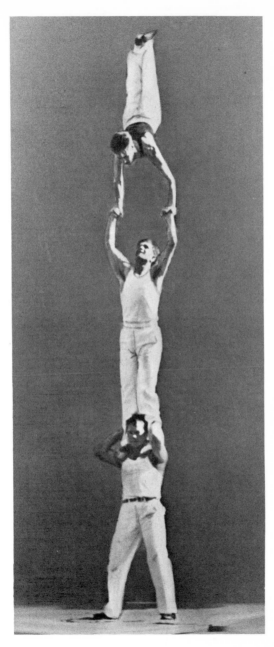

*Three high handstand, Dr. Martin on top - 1936*